Drug Resistance in Cancer
Mechanisms and Models

Drug resistance in cancer, whereby a proportion of cancer cells evades chemotherapy, poses a profound and continuing challenge for its effective treatment. The principles underlying the biological mechanisms behind this phenomenon are clearly explained in this volume. However, a deeper understanding of drug resistance requires a quantitative appreciation of the dynamic forces which shape tumour growth, including spontaneous mutation and selection processes. The authors seek to explain and to simplify these complex mechanisms, and to place them in a clinical context.

Clearly explained mathematical models are used to illustrate the biological principles and provide an insight into tumour development and the effectiveness and limitations of drug treatment. The book is suitable for those with a non-mathematical background and aims to enhance the effectiveness of cancer therapy. This is the firrt book to provide such an integrated account in a form accessible to the average doctor and scientist.

Drug Resistance in Cancer
Mechanisms and Models

J. H. GOLDIE
University of British Columbia
and
A. J. COLDMAN
British Columbia Cancer Agency

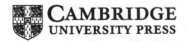

CAMBRIDGE UNIVERSITY PRESS
Cambridge, New York, Melbourne, Madrid, Cape Town, Singapore, São Paulo, Delhi

Cambridge University Press
The Edinburgh Building, Cambridge CB2 8RU, UK

Published in the United States of America by Cambridge University Press, New York

www.cambridge.org
Information on this title: www.cambridge.org/9780521111706

© Cambridge University Press 1998

This publication is in copyright. Subject to statutory exception
and to the provisions of relevant collective licensing agreements,
no reproduction of any part may take place without the written
permission of Cambridge University Press.

First published 1998
This digitally printed version 2009

A catalogue record for this publication is available from the British Library

Library of Congress Cataloguing in Publication data

Goldie, James H.

Drug resistance in cancer : models and mechanisms / J.H. Goldie
and A.J. Coldman.
  p. cm.
Includes bibliographical references.
ISBN 0 521 48273 9 (hardback)
1. Drug resistance in cancer cells.   2. Drug resistance in cancer
cells – Mathematical models.   I. Coldman, Andrew James, 1952– .
II. Title.
[DNLM: 1. Neoplasms – drug therapy.   2. Drug Resistance, Neoplasm.
QZ 267 G619d 1998]
RC271.C5G63 1998
616.99′4061–dc21   97-41916 CIP
Shared Cataloging for DNAL
Library of Congress

ISBN 978-0-521-48273-8 hardback
ISBN 978-0-521-11170-6 paperback

Every effort has been made in preparing this book to provide accurate and
up-to-date information which is in accord with accepted standards and
practice at the time of publication. Although case histories are drawn
from actual cases, every effort has been made to disguise the identities of
the individuals involved. Nevertheless, the authors, editors and publishers
can make no warranties that the information contained herein is totally
free from error, not least because clinical standards are constantly
changing through research and regulation. The authors, editors and
publishers therefore disclaim all liability for direct or consequential
damages resulting from the use of material contained in this book. Readers
are strongly advised to pay careful attention to information provided by
the manufacturer of any drugs or equipment that they plan to use.

Contents

Terms used in the book

α	mutation rate, spontaneous rate of resistance
b	birth rate
d	death rate
IC_{50}	concentration of drug required to inhibit cell growth by 50%
λ	growth rate
ρ	induced rate of resistance
$N(t)$	number of tumour cells
$P_0(N)$	probability of no resistance
$P_0(t)$ and P_c	probability of cure
$R(t)$	number of resistant cells at time t
$R_0, (R_0(t))$	resistant to no drugs (at time t)
$R_1 (R_1(t))$	resistant to drug 1 (at time t)
$R_2 (R_2(t))$	resistant to drug 2 (at time t)
$R_{12} (R_{12}(t))$	resistant to drugs 1 and 2 (at time t)
$S(t)$	number of sensitive cells
t	time
τ	doubling time

Preface

Drug resistance – the phenomenon whereby malignant tumours lose their responsiveness to therapeutic agents – is recognized as being the major obstacle to be overcome during the systemic therapy of cancer. In the 1980s and early 1990s an enormous amount of information was developed concerning the molecular mechanisms in the cell that can lead to resistance. In addition, these studies have provided insights into why resistance development is such a common property of cancer cells compared with normal cells.

We have been particularly interested in the processes that underlie the evolution of drug resistance within malignant cell populations and in the mathematical and biological models that have been developed to describe these processes. These models provide a greater intuitive understanding of drug resistance as well as providing insights into the more effective use of our available therapeutic agents.

Mathematical relationships in models may tell us little about specific mechanisms involved in various processes but they are often highly generalizable in terms of their inferences and usually lead to testable hypotheses.

Since we are concerned in this book with quantitative and mathematical models, any review of our own and related studies has to include some of the mathematics involved. The authors are aware of the reaction that is likely to engender in many readers (clinicians and biologists in particular) and the advice that was given to Professor Hawking ('Each equation in a book decreases its sales by half')[†] as well as the assessment of the schoolboy diarist and commentator, Nigel Molesworth ('All maths is friteful and mean 0, unless you are a grate brane')[‡]. We have

[†] Hawking, S.W. (1988). *A Brief History of Time*, p. vi. Bantam, Toronto.
[‡] Willans, G. and Searle, R. (1958). *The Compleet Molesworth*. Parrish, London.

accordingly attempted to keep the mathematical portions of the text as straightforward as possible, with largely algebraic relationshps discussed and only minimal amounts of calculus. We have avoided making reference to more rigorous developments utilizing techniques such as probability-generating functions and probability vectors, which will probably be inaccessible to most readers.

The mathematical relationships are accompanied by textual descriptions of the concepts being studied and we hope that this will aid in the development of an intuitive understanding of material.

JHG/AJC

1

The biological basis of cancer and the problem of drug resistance

1.1 Introduction

The phenomenon of resistance to environmental toxins has probably been present ever since life first evolved on earth. Any early living organism that happened to produce chemicals that were toxic to its competitors would have had a significant survival advantage in the struggle for existence. Competing species that failed to evolve a satisfactory protective mechanism against these toxins would have become extinct, but those that were able to circumvent successfully the toxins produced by other organisms would have been able to survive. Over the billions of years that life has evolved, organisms have developed an immense variety of chemical weapons against competitors and predators, who have in turn evolved mechanisms to permit their own survival.

The development of antibiotics and other chemical compounds for the treatment of infectious disease has been one of the triumphs of 20th century medicine. However, it is not clear at this point whether the gains made against many pathogenic organisms can be maintained. Strains of disease-producing bacteria that are resistant to most or even all of the available therapeutic agents are being increasingly encountered. The lay press is filled with stories about 'super bugs' that have 'learned' to overcome antibiotics. These popular accounts somehow manage to convey the picture of bacteria sitting down around a conference table and consciously planning their battle strategy against human beings. As if dealing with pathogenic microorganisms was not enough, the human race also has to contend with the evolution of its own aberrant cells, in the form of cancer, becoming resistant to the agents that are available for systemic treatment.

The underlying theme of this book is that there is a common thread to all of these problems. Namely, the capacity of all living organisms to produce genetically diverse individuals that differ in their ability to deal with various environmental insults. Increased capacity to deal with one type of insult may be associated with a diminished capacity to deal with others. Whether the net result is advantageous to the individual will depend on the nature of the environment that is imposing the selection pressure. In the case of pathogenic bacteria, the so-called 'super bugs' are probably not super at all but may well be less able to compete with their antibiotic-sensitive counterparts in the normal (i.e. relatively antibiotic-free) environment.

The development of chemical agents to treat cancer in the period since the Second World War has demonstrated that, firstly, only a proportion of types and individual cases of cancer can be considered highly sensitive to chemotherapeutic intervention and, secondly, virtually all types of cancer can evolve into a drug-resistant state.

It might be said that there are two broad viewpoints as to which are the most important determining factors in whether a malignant tumour will respond satisfactorily to drug treatment. The first viewpoint is basically that the sensitivity to drug treatment of a tumour results from a complex set of interacting phenomena. These include factors such as the pharmacology of the administered drugs and various attributes of the tumour itself and of the host organism. These factors would include the size and location of the tumour as well as its blood supply and growth rate. Other considerations would include the immune status of the host and the tolerance of the normal cells to the toxicity of the chemotherapy. This rather all-encompassing theory, which we might call 'epigenetic', is probably held by the majority of clinical oncologists and, in so far as it is based on valid measurements and reasonable assumptions, cannot be considered 'wrong' in any strict operational sense. We are using the term 'epigenetic' here in its rather older meaning of heritable adaptive changes in an organism that do not involve any actual alterations in DNA sequence or chromosomal configuration. Modern usage also tends to use epigenetic when describing alterations in DNA expression associated with changes with DNA methylation (see Chapter 8). The pragmatic question, however, is whether consideration of so many complex and interacting factors can readily yield practical therapeutic solutions.

A second viewpoint, to which the authors adhere, is that the primary basis for treatment resistance in cancer relates to the genetic diversity of the cancer cell population, which is, in turn, driven by a continuous series of mutations in a genetically unstable population. This so-called 'genetic' viewpoint is not really inconsistent with the epigenetic one, and the converse is also true. The question again comes down to certain pragmatic issues. Which of the myriad processes that appear to be operating within a cancer cell population are most likely to be responsible for therapeutic resistance and which of these are most likely to be vulnerable to effective intervention?

1.2   The beginnings of cancer chemotherapy

The first drugs that were found to have a consistent therapeutic effect against disseminated cancer were introduced into clinical practice in the 1940s. The studies by Gilman and colleagues in the USA utilizing a war gas derivative called nitrogen mustard represented the first time that an organic chemical was shown to have an unambiguous therapeutic effect against at least one type of cancer.

The patient treated in these studies had an advanced malignant lymphoma and experienced significant regression of disease after the first treatment. Because of the toxicity associated with the treatment, the second course of therapy was given at a reduced dose with an associated lesser therapeutic effect. By the time the third treatment was given, the tumour no longer responded to the chemotherapeutic agent. This first systematic effort to utilize chemical anticancer compounds not only demonstrated the capacity of the agents to produce a major effect against the tumour but also was associated with the first demonstration of clinical resistance occurring during treatment. About the same time as these studies, Haddow in England reported on the antitumour properties of the drug urethane, which was shown to have some beneficial effects in chronic myelogenous leukaemia and myeloma.

Shortly after the above studies were reported, Farber in Boston utilized the folic acid antagonist aminopterin to treat acute childhood leukaemia. The decision to use this drug was based in part on the observation that the use of the vitamin folic acid appeared actually to aggravate the course of the disease, suggesting that blocking folic acid metabolism might be beneficial. In a number of these patients treated with aminopterin, significant clinical and haematological improvement was noted. Unfortunately, within a short time of discontinuance of the treatment the bone marrow again reverted to a leukaemic state. Repeat applications of the chemotherapy tended to produce only short-lived responses followed ultimately by complete refractoriness to further therapy.

Reading the literature of the time, it is apparent that clinicians did not have a clear picture of what was actually occurring to the patients' disease under the impact of chemotherapy. Although there was awareness that cancer cells were being killed off or dying, there was also the impression that the antitumour agent was in some way correcting a metabolic abnormality in the cancer cells and temporarily restoring the marrow to normal function. The analogy with megaloblastic anaemia being treated with vitamin B_{12} was thought to be relevant. It would take a number of years of experimental study to delineate better the processes that occurred when malignancies were being treated by anti-cancer compounds. As will be described below, it was not until the early 1960s that a really useful model of cancer chemotherapy came to be developed.

These early examples that it was possible to produce significant regressions of certain types of cancer with a variety of pharmacological agents served to generate great optimism that successful treatment of metastatic cancer was a realistic goal. It is apparent now, however, that despite more than half a century of determined effort many obstacles remain to achieving therapeutic results comparable to those accomplished in the treatment of bacterial infection. There have been some gratifying advances made in the therapy of a number of specific types of malignancy, particularly those of the paediatric age group as well as germ cell tumours and malignant lymphomas, but the sober fact remains that many of the malignancies of middle and older life remain incurable once they have extended beyond the point where local forms of therapy can be applied.

In this text, we will explore some of the general processes that appear to underlie the cancer cell's capacity to display resistance to virtually all of the therapeutic agents that may be directed against it. We will review a number of the theories that have been put forward to explain this phenomenon and will, in particular, give emphasis to the role that heritable genetic changes (mutations) in the individual cells may have in contributing to resistance.

1.3   The genetic origins of cancer

Since the 1980s, an enormous amount of information has been generated regarding the molecular changes that occur when a normal cell is transformed into a malignant one. A comprehensive biological model for the origin of cancer is emerging and it is becoming clearer why the development of drug resistance is such a fundamental component of the behaviour of malignant cell populations.

Cancer can be defined as a disease arising when a single cell, through changes in the expression of its genetic material, acquires the property of excess proliferation over that which is required for maintenance of physiological cell numbers. Associated with this change are progressive losses of normal function and the acquisition of properties such as *invasiveness*, whereby the cancer cells infiltrate into the surrounding normal tissues, and *metastasis*, where the cancer cell is able to enter the systemic circulation and set up sites of secondary growth in distant regions of the body. Although small numbers of cancer cells will have no ill effects on the patient, the relentless increase in the size of the malignant population will cause progressive dysfunction until death results. With the exception of the very rare instances when cancer spontaneously regresses, a malignancy is invariably fatal in the absence of effective treatment .

Many of the genetic changes that result in the development and progression of cancer appear to result from *mutations*, which may be defined as heritable alterations in the cell's genetic information. The heritable nature of mutations is a key factor in the production of cancer, and mutations are to be distinguished from changes in cell function that are not heritable and hence are not passed on from one cell generation to the next.

1.4   Mutations

Mutations may be considered as falling into two main broad categories:

1. *Genetic mutations.* This term refers to changes in the sequence of base pairs in the DNA molecule itself. This can affect the structural gene, resulting in an abnormal protein, or can affect the DNA sequences that control gene expression. Examples would include point, frameshift and missense mutations.
2. *Chromosomal mutations.* These can be defined as 'any structural change involving the gain, loss or relocation of chromosome segments' (German, 1983) and may be microscopic or submicroscopic. They may include deletions, duplications and inversions of short segments of chromosomes. Whole chromosomes may be involved,

which will result in gain or loss in the total number of chromosomes in the cell.

A type of chromosomal mutation common in cancer is *gene amplification* whereby the number of copies of a gene are increased, often in an expanded region of the chromosome that is called a *homogeneously staining region* (HSR). Related to HSRs are small chromosomal fragments called *double minutes* (DMs), which may contain amplified gene segments. Translocation of one part of a chromosome to another entirely different chromosome is frequently seen in various cancers, particularly those of the lymphatic or haematopoietic systems. This may result in continuous overproduction of a growth-controlling protein. Genetic mutations are seen in both neoplastic and nonneoplastic cells, but chromosomal mutations are rare in nonneoplastic cells.

Germ-line mutations refer to mutations occurring within the sexual cells (gametes) of a multicellular organism and which, therefore, can be passed on to the cells of that organism's progeny. *Somatic mutations* are those that occur in the nonsexual cells of the body and since they do not affect the germ-line they cannot be inherited by offspring. Although some cancers are associated with germ-line mutations, the great majority appear to arise through mutations in somatic cells.

Spontaneous mutations are those that occur with a certain low frequency in the germ and somatic cells and for which there are no obvious initiating factors. *Induced mutations* are associated with a higher frequency than spontaneous mutations and can be brought about through the effect of a variety of mutagenic agents (chemicals, ionizing radiation). A key element with respect to describing mutations is that whatever their inherent frequency they are random in nature; that is, whether the mutation occurs or not is inherently unpredictable even if the probability of it occurring can be estimated. (Spontaneous mutations are to be distinguished from directed mutations, which imply that an environmental agent induces a mutation that is specific to itself in a Lamarckian sense as opposed to a Darwinian one. This topic will be discussed in detail in Chapters 4 and 8.) It should be remembered that the rarity of an event occurring is not evidence that it is random. Lunar eclipses, triple conjunctions of the planets, etc. are infrequent events, but their occurrence can be predicted with great accuracy. Predictable phenomena are referred to as *deterministic*. If we had a die with six dots on five of its sides and one dot on the remaining side then the number six would come up with a high frequency (five out of six tosses), but it would still not be possible to predict what number would arise at the next toss. We can only estimate the probability of it being six or one. Random outcomes are called *stochastic* events, and a series of stochastic events is called a stochastic process. Mutations are examples of stochastic events and the number of mutations in a growing population is a stochastic process.

We have mentioned that spontaneous mutations are rare events. Typically we find the probability of the change in any one gene occurring is in the order of 1 in 10^6 to 1 in 10^8. That is, we would say that the mutation rate or probability is 10^{-6} to 10^{-8} per cell generation. Mutation *frequency* is usually meant in the sense of the frequency of occurrence of mutants in a population.

An interesting question is why do the mutation rates in human cells (and mammalian systems generally) assume the value that they do. A possible explanation for this has been suggested by the studies of Manfred Eigen (Eigen, 1992), who has examined the processes that may have been involved in the formation of life on earth. Eigen has looked at the mutation rates that occur within viruses and has noted a relationship between the observed rate and the information content of the viruses' genetic material. This requires determining just how much information is present within the genetic code of an organism.

In 1948, Claude Shannon working at the Bell laboratories in the USA developed a mathematical theory for describing the information content of a message and for how the message could be coded and decoded during transmission. Although Shannon was initially looking at the problem of electronic transmission of language messages, it was apparent that the mathematical formulation, known as *information theory*, could be applied to a great range of phenomena in which a coded message of any kind undergoes transmission. In Shannon's approach, the information content of a message was determined by the number of yes/no answers that would be required to specify exactly the sequence of designated symbols in a message of any arbitrary length. It is convenient to express the number of yes/no answers in logarithms to the base 2.

We start with a number of symbols (letters in the case of a human language, nucleotide bases in the case of DNA) and a message of N symbols in length. In the case of human DNA we have four symbols (adenine, guanine, cytosine and thymidine) and a message that contains approximately 3×10^9 base pairs. The information content is $4^{3\times10/9} = 2^{2\times3\times10/9}$; from this the $\log_2 = 6 \times 10^9$, which is defined as the information content in binary digits (bits) (this assumes that there is little redundancy in the code, i.e. that a single base-pair change can alter the meaning of the message). Eigen found that the mutation rate in viruses was inversely proportional to the information content of the viral nucleic acid, i.e. $1/N$. He hypothesized that the tolerable rate for making mistakes per transmission of a message of N length must be no more than $1/N$ where N is the information content in bits. Eigen refers to the value of $1/N$ as the error threshold. The term error threshold as used here is different in meaning from the term usually employed in classical information theory. It might be better described as the 'biological error threshold' above which the error probability will produce excessive numbers of genetic mistakes. If the error rate for duplicating the message is equal to or greater than $1/N$ then there would be at least one mistake per duplication, which would result in progressive degradation of the message content. Error rates higher than $1/N$ would result in what Eigen calls an 'error catastrophe', which would soon render the organism nonviable.

It has been estimated that the frequency of single base-pair changes in human DNA is in the order of 10^{-10} per cell generation. Since the message for a typical protein contains between 10^3 and 10^4 base pairs, we can see that the error threshold for a typical protein turns out to be one mistake per 10^6 to 10^7 duplications. This value is approximately equal to the average mutation rate observed in human systems.[†] It suggests, therefore, that nature normally operates the mutation rate at just below the error threshold for the system. This permits just enough genetic variation to give the species adaptability without allowing the genetic message to become seriously degraded.

1.5   Oncogenes and tumour suppressor genes

There are two main types of gene that have critical importance in the control of cell division and in the development of cancer. The first

[†] A mutation of 10^{-5} or 10^{-7} represents the average for the system. There are a few places in the genome where mutation rates significantly higher than this occur. One such location is where the variable region of the immunoglobulin molecule is coded. Mutation rates in the order of 10^{-4} are observed here. As the generation of antibody diversity has a powerful survival value, evolution has favoured high mutation rates in this discrete area.

Certain types of chromosomal mutation (gene amplification), which are seen in tumour cells but not normal cells, have mutation rates as high as 10^{-3} per cell generation. Not all genes appear to be susceptible to being amplified in this manner as the effect is seen only at certain points in the chromosomes (areas of higher instability?). Certain oncogenes and some of the genes that mediate drug resistance are frequently amplified in cancer cells.

group of genes, oncogenes, appear to be primarily involved in providing positive growth signals to the cell in response to a variety of internal and external cellular stimuli. Many of the oncogenes are key components of the pathways from the cell surface to the nucleus. Many growth factors and certain hormones utilize these pathways for providing stimuli to the cell nucleus, a process described as signal transduction. The normally functioning oncogene ('cancer gene') is usually referred to as a proto-oncogene, suggesting that it has the capacity, after mutation, of functioning as a cancer-inducing gene. These names are embedded in the literature now, but they are rather misleading, suggesting that a malign providence placed the genes there for the express purpose of producing cancer. The oncogenes are, in fact, vitally important growth regulatory genes whose significance is attested by the fact that they have been conserved through the process of evolution from protozoa to humans. We do not refer to the kidneys as 'the uraemia-producing organs' and the term 'oncogene' does carry a sinister connotation.

The other major group of genes involved in the control of cell division is usually called anti-oncogenes or tumour suppressor genes. These genes basically function antagonistically to the oncogenes, producing a brake to the proliferative impetus they provide. There may be as many as 50–100 oncogenes and anti-oncogenes acting in concert to regulate the movement of cells through the cell cycle (q.v.). Some genes are more important in particular tissues than others, and some appear to be more frequently involved in neoplastic transformation.

In addition to regulating events in the cell cycle, some of the tumour suppressor genes play a key role in causing cells to undergo differentiation or actual dissolution. Increasingly, the view is being expressed by many authors that in multicell organisms cells are programmed to die off unless they receive a positive signal to continue dividing. Loss of the ability to undergo cell death under the appropriate conditions, combined with an abnormal growth signal, may constitute the fundamental basis of the cancerous state.

1.6   Genetic instability and cancer

In 1976 Nowell postulated that cancers were 'genetically unstable' compared with normal cells and over time would accumulate mutations that would result in cells with progressively more abnormal properties. This would include the capacity to invade surrounding tissues and to establish distant secondary colonies. Any mutation that conferred a slight growth advantage would be favoured and retention of normal function would not necessarily be advantageous.

Abundant evidence has tended to confirm this model of cancer development, with many of the molecular events associated with neoplastic transformation being identified. As suggested by Loeb (1991) it would appear that the first step in carcinogenesis may be a mutation that results in a so-called mutator phenotype. This phenotype is characterized by a mutation in one of the genes that is responsible for the fidelity of genetic replication. This will render the cell prone to further mutations, which can result in progressive loss of constraints on cell proliferation and sensitivity to normal growth-regulating signals. The result will be a rapidly expanding population of cells in which progressively more malignant phenotypes will be produced. This mutation cascade will typically occur as a series of somatic mutations in cells that still have some stem cell capacity (see Chapter 2). If the initial mutation occurs in the individual's germ cells, then the progeny of that individual will have the mutation present in all of their somatic cells and will be at great risk for subsequent development of cancer.

One of the important genetic elements that influences the probability of cancer developing is the *p53 gene*, one of the tumour suppressor genes. The protein produced by this gene regulates the movement of cells through the cell cycle and initiates a type of check programme for abnormalities in DNA structure. Errors in the genetic code are identified and corrected through activation of one of the DNA repair systems.

If there has been more damage to the integrity of the DNA than can be readily repaired, the p53 gene signals a cell self-destruction programme to commence. This is known as *programmed cell death* or *apoptosis* (Chapter 3). The gene p53 functions either to repair mutated DNA or, if the damage is too severe, to destroy the cell rather than have it retained within the system. Mutated cells are thus culled from the population so that the stability of the genetic message in the normal cells is maintained. A mutation affecting p53 will thus greatly increase the cell's propensity for undergoing further mutations. Although there are two gene copies (alleles) for p53 normally present, mutation in one of the alleles can result in loss of p53 function (a so-called dominant-negative mutation) through the mutant p53 protein binding to the normal p53 and preventing it from functioning. It has been estimated that more than 50% of all instances of human cancer are associated with mutations in p53, suggesting its vital role in normal growth and differentiation. Inheritance of a defective p53 gene results in a genetic disorder (Li-Fraumeni syndrome) in which there is a greatly increased incidence of a variety of cancers, particularly breast cancer. Although defective p53 on its own will not necessarily result in malignancy, when combined with mutations altering the function of one of the positive growth signalling genes (cellular oncogene), the cell will have gone a long distance towards acquiring a malignant phenotype. There are other genes that may function somewhat similarly to that for p53, but p53 appears to be particularly important with respect to neoplastic transformation.

Although spontaneous or induced mutations appear to be involved with most forms of human cancer, certain viruses are strongly suggested as playing a role in the aetiology of certain types of malignancy. In many animal species, viruses are a common contributing element in cancer causation (in some species perhaps the most common). In these cases, the virus may actually insert a mutated oncogene into the cell's DNA or insert an abnormal controlling gene adjacent to a normal cellular oncogene. The effect is very much as if the cellular gene itself had undergone a mutation. At least three common human viruses are thought to be important in cancer causation. These are the human papilloma virus (HPV) in cervical cancer, Epstein–Barr virus (EBV) in nasopharyngeal cancer and in Burkitt's lymphoma and the hepatitis B virus (HBV) in hepatocellular carcinoma. These three viruses are all DNA viruses and it has been found that they all are capable of producing a protein that binds to and inactivates the p53 protein or opposes p53 function indirectly. This clearly could play a significant role in generating malignancy. However, viruses have not been implicated in the majority of types of human cancer.

It is worthwhile pointing out that while cancer is considered a common disease in our society, it is in fact the result of an extremely rare event. As it is, about 3/4 of our population do not develop clinical malignancy in their lifetime. It has been estimated that the cells in a human being will, over the course of a lifetime, produce an aggregate total one quintillion (10^{15}) divisions. As we will see, it only takes *one* of these progressing to become malignant to produce the clinical condition of cancer. In contrast, all organs of the body can tolerate the deaths of millions (even billions) of cells and still maintain vital function. It is apparent that complex multicellular organisms are constructed in such a way as to control cell proliferation rigorously, and, as has been said, 'the default mode of the cell is to die out'.

How many different types of cancer are there likely to be? Traditional histopathological classifications generally yield about 200–400 varieties. The information being gained regarding the molecular genotypes that may exist suggests a far greater number. We can calculate a very rough estimate (which may be out by many orders of magnitude) by simply calculating the permutations that may exist with the known or estimated genetic possibilities. We begin by taking the lower estimate of the number of oncogenes and anti-oncogenes (50) and assume that they all have the capacity to contribute to the neoplastic state. Depending on the type of cancer it seems that between two and ten mutant genes are required for transformation. If we assume the average is six, then we can estimate the number of permutations of six that will be present for any six of these genes. The number of permutations of the oncogenes drawn from a population of 50 is equal to $50!/40! \div 6!$. Which is approximately 11×10^9. However, there appear to be many mutant forms that can exist for many of the cancer-associated genes. If we assume a low number (say ten) mutant forms for each gene, then the potential number of cancer genotypes becomes $10^{11 \times 10^9}$, a number so staggeringly large as to defy comprehension. Of course, in reality many genotypes may be 'forbidden' in the sense that they are nonviable, and some genetic mutations will occur with much greater frequency than others. Even so, the potential genetic variety of cancers must be forbiddingly large.

1.7   The relationship between drug resistance and the neoplastic state

One of the puzzling things about drug resistance is that it almost invariably occurs when dealing with neoplastic cells but it is virtually never seen with normal cell systems. If anything, the tolerance to chemotherapy of the normal cell systems often declines with time, possibly owing to stem cell depletion. About the only circumstance where something resembling drug resistance in normal cells occurs is with regard to hair follicle cells in patients. Many antineoplastic agents cause varying degrees of baldness; this is produced by temporary interruptions in the hair follicle growth that results in a hair shaft that is thinner and weaker than normal. When the hair shaft grows above the surface of the scalp it readily breaks off leaving the patient 'bald'. Once treatment is stopped normal hair growth resumes.

Occasionally hair growth will resume in a patient who is still on chemotherapy, suggesting that the follicles have become resistant to the drug. Although it is not certain why hair growth commences in these patients, the phenomenon lacks some of the features that are seen with drug resistance. For one thing, the renewed hair growth tends to be uniform over the whole scalp (and not patchy, which would suggest genetic variance in individual follicle cells) and the baldness will recur if chemotherapy is restarted after a time off therapy. Since this appears to be a type of variable response that is characterized by individual patients, it may simply suggest that some people are constitutively less sensitive to the hair follicle toxicity produced by chemotherapy.

Immunosuppressive drugs (some of which are antineoplastic agents as well) can be given to suppress the growth of normal immune cells for, in some instances, many years without resistance appearing. Certain immunological diseases (such as Wegener's granulomatosis and periarteritis nodosa) that appear to be in the borderland between the normal state and malignancy will display resistance to treatment but generally only after extended periods of treatment. It is apparent, therefore, that the acquisition of drug resistance can be considered to be one of the properties of cancer along with the more usually recognized properties of unrestrained growth, invasion and metastasis.

The relationship between drug resistance and malignancy is partly owing to the fact that permitting mutations to accumulate in dividing cells will increase the probability that there will be mutations directly affecting the proteins involved with mediating drug action. Both cancer (unrestrained growth) and drug resistance (tolerance of genetic damage, molecular heterogeneity) are seen to be consequences of a primary genetic instability.

1.8 Methods for measuring drug response in experimental systems

There are two usual methods of estimating drug sensitivity. The first of these involves counting the total number of intact cells in a standard volume of fluid and comparing this with the number of cells present in the same volume of fluid after exposure to a drug. The untreated cells will increase in number at their own specific growth rate and we can estimate the drug concentration required to inhibit the treated cells to 50% of the number reached by the unexposed cells after a fixed period of time (e.g. 24 hours, 48 hours). This concentration is called the IC_{50} (concentration of drug required to inhibit cell growth by 50%). As the cell line becomes more resistant, the IC_{50} value will progressively increase.

The IC_{50} method is technically easy to perform and is reproducible, but it does not provide direct information as to how many cells are killed by a particular drug exposure. This type of information is better obtained from a second technique called *dose response curve*, in which a cell population is exposed to a specific *concentration × time factor of drug* ($c \times t$) (Fig. 1.1). Following drug exposure, the cells are grown in a semisolid medium in a dispersed state. A known number of cells are cultured in the dispersed form and the growth of each viable individual cell can be detected as a discrete colony of cells. Cells that have survived the drug exposure will continue to proliferate and if they undergo sufficient sequential divisions to produce 64 cells or more the cell will be counted as viable. The number of cells capable of giving rise to colonies is counted for each concentration of drug so that a graph of number of colonies versus increasing dose is constructed.

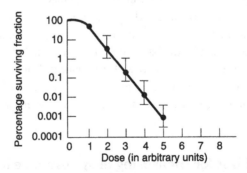

Fig. 1.1. Hypothetical dose–response curve with percentage surviving colonies plotted against increasing dose. Each measured point on the curve shows the mean and standard duration of multiple replicate assays. There is often a small 'shoulder' in the early part of the curve indicating a subtoxic dose of drug at the lowest dose used.

Not all of the intact and apparently viable cells present in the tumour or cell culture will have the capacity to undergo several sequential divisions. Therefore, it is necessary to estimate the colony-forming efficiency of the untreated cells to compare with the colony-forming efficiency of the treated population. A known number of untreated cells are plated out into culture and the numbers of colonies counted. The ratio of number of colonies over total number of cells plated times 100% gives the colony-forming efficiency of the cell population. The value for the colony-forming efficiency of the untreated cells can be set as equal to 100% and the values for the cells treated at increasing drug concentration are then plotted on a graph to produce the dose response curve. It is convenient to represent values for colony-forming efficiency on a logarithmic scale and dose on either a logarithmic or an arithmetic scale. There are some important advantages to colony-forming assays. If there are relatively few cells in the target population that are capable of division, then it is important to determine this fact to ensure that the treated populations are scaled against the colony-forming efficiency of the untreated cells. As well, the test of whether a cell can undergo several rounds of division is a very stringent one for viability that has special relevance to cancer chemotherapy.

The problem with colony assays is that they are labour intensive, require special culture conditions that will permit dispersed cells to grow and they take usually 7 to 10 days to complete. However, if a particular tumour cell line is known to have a very high colony-forming efficiency (50–100%) and if it is found that treated cells undergo rapid physical dissolution, then simply counting cells directly after drug exposure may yield information similar to that produced by a colony-forming assay.

1.9   The log kill law

If the colony-forming efficiency of the untreated cells is (for example) 100% and the total cell population we are examining consists of 10^6 cells, we can count the number of colony-forming cells present after a given dose of drug. We might find that only 1% of the treated cells survived (10^4), which means that 99% of the cells were killed. If a second dose of drug, the same as the first, is given to the population of cells when it is at the level of 10^4 then we would find that again 99% of the cells are killed resulting in 10^2 viable cells being left. If the same dose of drug is given over a range of numbers of tumour cells, we would find that the same dose always kills the same fraction of cells but the absolute number of cells killed will depend on the number of cells present at the time the treatment was given. In this sense, it does not become any 'easier' to kill smaller numbers of cells.

A 1% survival is equivalent to saying that there was a 0.01 probability of any individual cell surviving. The negative logarithm of 0.01 is 2, and this is referred to as the log kill of the drug against the cells and indicates that the number of viable cells was reduced by two logarithmic decades. If a larger dose of drug is used and this reduces the probability of cell survival to 0.0001 then this is described as a four log kill, etc. This is convenient terminology to use in chemotherapy experiments where it is usual to observe the killing of a large proportion of the treated malignant cells.

This relationship between administered dose (D) and cell survival probability (P) is referred to as the *log kill law*. It can be stated as the log probability of survival varies with dose or in symbols:

$$\log(P_s) = -\beta D,$$

where β is the constant of cell killing, a number which will vary for different drugs and different cell lines; it is the slope of the cell killing curve.

If the dose of drug is doubled ($2D$) then the probability of cell survival is now equal to the square of the probability of survival at dose D, i.e. P_s^2:

$$-\beta 2D = 2\log(P_s) = \log(P_s^2).$$

This relationship can be easily understood by simply imagining an experiment where the initial dose, D, produces a cell survival probability of 0.01. If a second dose is given immediately after the first (before any cell regrowth occurs) then the residual population will be reduced by another two logs (since it is known that the same dose always kills the same fraction of cells). The final cell survival probability will, therefore, be $0.01 \times 0.01 = 0.0001. = 0.01^2$.

The physical basis for the log kill law was outlined by Wilcox in 1963 (see discussion by Skipper (1980)). The killing of a cell by a drug is essentially a chemical reaction and, therefore, would be expected to follow the laws of solution thermodynamics. In any solution of drug molecules, a small fraction of the molecules will have a much greater than average kinetic energy associated with them. It will be these molecules that will be sufficiently energetic to interact with key molecular targets within a cell. In addition to having sufficient energy, the drug molecule will also have to be oriented the the right way at the time of drug–target interaction and there will be varying degrees of chemical affinity between the drug and target. Therefore, the critical cell killing interaction is a stochastic event and can be described by probability theory. We can increase the cell killing effect either by increasing the concentration of drug molecules (giving a larger dose) or by increasing the number of molecules that have a greater kinetic energy (by heating the system). Where there is a direct linear relationship between the probability of cell killing and the concentration of drug, this is described as a *first-order kinetic reaction.*

Virtually all of the standard chemotherapeutic agents start to exert significant cell killing effects on sensitive tumour cells at concentrations ranging from 10^{-8} to 10^{-6} M. It has been estimated that it generally requires from 10^3 to 10^5 drug molecules to gain entry to the cell to produce lethal damage. This can be contrasted with the properties of the extraordinarily toxic plant glycoprotein ricin, for which only one to two molecules per cell is sufficient to produce lethal injury.

1.10   Definitions of drug resistance

The terms drug resistance and sensitivity are relative conditions that, to be meaningful, must be defined with respect to some standard reference frame. In addition, the drug-resistant state needs to refer to a specific drug and a particular concentration and duration of exposure to that drug. Where the resistant cells have been produced by drug exposure of a wild or sensitive cell line then the degree of resistance of the derived cells will be referred back to that of the initial sensitive cell population. The 'wild' or parent cell line refers to the dominant phenotype observed prior to selection by a toxic substance. This will be the cell type best suited for survival under the initial conditions. It should be borne in mind that *all* conditions are selecting, including the initial environment in which the cancer cell formed. Exposure to a toxic agent changes the environment and now selects for a different phenotype.

It is relatively easy to define the conditions for resistance in experimental systems. Typically, if we wish to produce a drug-resistant cell line in a tissue culture system, the initial sensitive cells can be exposed to

increasing concentrations of drug. Over time, the behaviour of the treated cell population will begin to change and after initial signs of growth
retardation the tumour cells will become capable of proliferating continuously in drug concentrations that were initially effective in producing
cell death (Fig. 1.2). When such a cell line is cultured in the absence of
the cytotoxic agent that was used to produce the resistance, it will generally retain its degree of resistance for an extended period of time. In
some circumstances, however, the cell line will progressively reduce its
degree of resistance and revert back to its initial drug-sensitive state. The
first circumstance where the resistance is maintained for an extended
period is described as a condition of *stable* resistance; where resistance
is progressively lost, it is *unstable* resistance. Further it is common to
observe that cells which are resistant to one concentration of a drug may
be sensitive to higher concentrations of the same drug. If a cell is completely resistant to inhibition by a particular drug concentration we can
then say in mathematical terms that the probability of the cell surviving
exposure to the drug equals 1. This would define a state of *complete*
resistance. However, if the probability of the cell surviving is less than
one, but greater than that for the wild type then we refer to these states
as being ones of *partial* resistance.

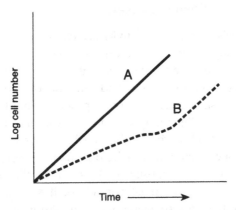

Fig. 1.2. Plots of growth curves of tumour cells in tissue culture. A. Untreated
control cells. B. Cells exposed to continuous concentrations of a cytotoxic
drug. Growth curve initially slows then recovers, becoming parallel to that of
control cells. At this point a drug-resistant line has manifested itself. The
process can then be repeated any arbitrary number of times to produce a
progressively more resistant line.

To simplify many of the mathematical developments describing drug resistance it is often convenient to consider a cell's probability of survival as being either 1 (complete resistance) or 0 (complete sensitivity). This is obviously an oversimplification and we can assume that in real cellular systems there is a tremendous range of cell survival probabilities lying between the two extremes. It is the average, or mean, cell survival probability that will tend to define the degree of drug resistance of the population as a whole.

1.11 Estimations of relative drug resistance by dose response curves

Figure 1.3 shows three theoretical survival curves expressed on a log–log scale. Curve A represents the curve for the wild-type cells, which are the most sensitive. Curve B represents a survival curve of an intermediate-level resistant line and curve C that of a highly resistant population. If we were only to consider the dose needed to generate the same log kill in each cell line, we can see that it takes three times the dose to produce the same five log kill in B compared with A. Using this comparison, line

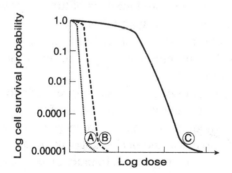

Fig. 1.3. Three hypothetical dose response curves (log surviving function plotted against log dose). A is the mild or sensitive cell line, B is moderately resistant and C highly resistant. Depending on whether we use as our measure of resistance the dose required to produce an equivalent log kill in each cell line or whether we use the dose required to produce (for example) a five log kill in A and measure that dose in B and C, we will see different quantitative estimates of the relative resistance of each line (see text). (Reproduced, from Goldie, J.H. and Ling, V. (1992), with the kind permission of Rodar Publication, Montreal, Canada.)

B is three times more resistant than A. If instead, we look at the dose required to produce a five log kill in A and then assess that dose against B, we observe that only one log kill has been produced. We can, therefore, state that by this measure line B is 10 000 times more resistant than A. This degree of difference would translate into a marked effect at the clinical level and yet might be associated with only small differences in the biochemical constitution of the two cell types. The difference might, in fact, be too small to be readily detected by the usual analytic means. Cell line C is very highly resistant to drug by any standard of measure. It will require hundreds of times the dose of drug to produce an equivalent five log kill in line C compared with A. Likewise, the dose that will produce a five log kill in line A has virtually no effect on C.

Cell lines such as C can be readily produced in *in vitro* experimental systems and will probably display marked molecular changes compared with sensitive cells. However, less-resistant cells such as B may be more likely to be the type seen clinically.

1.12 Definitions of clinical sensitivity and resistance

When we come to define what constitutes clinical resistance to cancer chemotherapy, the circumstances are more complex. We generally have to use gross measurements and markers of tumour presence within the patient. These include physical and radiological assessments of tumour size. It may also be possible to include biochemical measurements of some tumour index substance that is present in the serum and can be assayed quantitatively.

In principle, a tumour can be considered sensitive to chemotherapy if the number of tumour cells killed per course of treatment is greater than the amount of tumour regrowth that occurs prior to the next course of therapy. We refer to this as the *net* log kill of the treatment (initial log kill minus amount of tumour regrowth). In practical terms, however, this net decrease must be sufficiently great to translate into significant overall reduction in tumour mass and, therefore, be associated with clinical benefit.

The usual lowest category of tumour response is designated a *partial response* and is defined as a 50% reduction in tumour mass (with no associated increase in any known site of disease) for at least 1 month's duration. A *complete response* represents the disappearance of all detectable signs of malignancy for at least 1 month. Lesser categories of response may be noted, such as <50% reduction in tumour mass or cessation of measurable tumour growth. Although those effects are usually not considered of sufficient magnitude to constitute useful clinical sensitivity, if they are sustained for a substantial period of time (i.e. several months) they can represent clinical benefit to the patients. Such effects are categorized as *minor responses* or *disease stabilization*. These descriptions are obviously phenomenological terms that give only the crudest impression of what is actually happening within the tumour. Changes in tumour volume obviously represent the net balance between cell killing, rate of cell dissolution and cell regrowth and will tend to underestimate significantly the actual numbers of tumour cells that are being killed by each application of treatment.

If a complete remission lasts indefinitely with no evidence of tumour recurrence and with the patient (or animal) living a normal life expectancy, then this can be considered to constitute a clinical cure. The presumption is that all of the tumour cells have been killed by the treatment or at least reduced to a low number and are incapable of growing back to reconstitute the clinical disease.

Clinical resistance is a term that tends to be used somewhat loosely but is usually taken to refer to a progressive increase in tumour mass despite continued treatment. If a malignancy displays resistance to chemotherapy right from the outset of treatment, this is usually termed *intrinsic resistance*, implying an innate resistance property of the cells. If the tumour is initially sensitive to chemotherapy and then commences regrowth despite ongoing treatment, then this is referred to as *acquired resistance*, suggesting the acquisition of new properties by the tumour. Since clinical response will be dictated, in part, by the initial *proportion* of resistant cells, a clear-cut distinction between these two states may not be possible.

1.13   Summary and conclusions

We have briefly reviewed the development of cancer chemotherapy, discussed some of the methods used for measuring anticancer drug effects in experimental systems and have introduced the concept of drug resistance. A cancer cell population may display progressive diminution in drug sensitivity (acquired drug resistance) or may at the outset exhibit insufficient sensitivity to treatment that tolerated doses of chemotherapy will be ineffectual in producing clinical benefit (intrinsic resistance). Following the early pioneering efforts in cancer chemotherapy, a major effort was undertaken during the 1960s to understand the reasons for success or failure in cancer chemotherapy better. The methodologies that were developed to study this problem will be discussed in the next chapter.

References

Eigen, M. (1992). *Steps Towards Life*. Oxford University Press, Oxford. An account of the basic chemical processes that may have led to the formation of life on earth. It contains many interesting examples as to how genetic information can be stored, modified and transmitted. The book deals with a number of abstract theoretical and mathematical concepts as they apply to molecular evolution, but the author does not employ much in the way of mathematical formulae; rather he relies on verbal examples and well executed diagrams to illustrate the concepts.

German, J. (1983). In *Chromosome Mutation and Neoplasia*, ed. J. German, pp. xv–xxv. Alan R. Liss, New York, quoting Reiger R., Michaels A. and Green M. (1979). In *Glossary of Genetics and Cytogenetics*, 4th edn, p. 98. Springer Verlag, New York.

Goldie, J.H. and Ling, V. (1992). The evolution of drug resistance. *Can. J. Oncol.*, 1, 1–15.

Loeb, L. (1991). Mutator phenotype may be required for multi-stage carcinogenesis. *Cancer Res.*, 51: 3075–3079.

Nowell, P.C. (1976). The clonal evolution of tumour cell populations. *Science*, 194: 23–28.

Shannon, C. (1948). A mathematical theory of communication. *Bell Syst. Tech. J.*, 27, 379–423, 623–56. The classic paper in information theory, which is directed toward a specialist readership.

Skipper, H.E. (1980). Some thoughts regarding the modes of action of drugs on cells and/or application of available pharmacokinetic data. In *Cancer Chemotherapy*, Vol. 10. University Microfilms International, Ann Arbor, MI. This book is part of a series of texts published by the author in which he summarized his vast experience in the field of experimental chemotherapy. The text is well written and illustrated with abundant examples of the author's own experimental data.

Further reading

Brison, O. (1993). Gene amplification and tumor progression. *Biochim. Biophys. Acta*, 1155: 25–41.

Brock, D.J. (1993). *Molecular Genetics for the Clinician*. Cambridge University Press, Cambridge. A short but comprehensive introduction to those aspects of molecular genetics that appear to be of special clinical relevance. The sections on genetic diseases and chromosomal mapping are particularly useful.

Cheng, K.C. and Loeb, L.A. (1993). Genomic instability and tumour progression. Mechanistic considerations. *Adv. Cancer Res.*, 60: 121–156.

Greenblatt, M.S., Bennett, W.P. Hollstein, M. *et al.* (1994). Mutations in the p53 tumour suppressor gene. Clues to cancer etiology and molecular pathogenesis. *Cancer Res.*, 54: 4855–4878.

Griswold, D.P. (1990). Scientific basis for multicombination chemotherapy. In *Proc. 5th Ngoya Symp. Cancer Treatment*, ed. K. Kimura *et al.* Excerpta Medico, Amsterdam.

Harris, A. (1992). p.53 expression in human breast cancer. *Adv. Cancer Res.*, 59: 69–88.

Lewin, B. (1995). *Gene V.* Wiley, New York. A comprehensive and up-to-date text dealing with all the various aspects of molecular biology. The text is lavishly illustrated and written in an almost conversational style. The author has achieved the feat of being able to reverse the trend in large text books towards ever smaller print and more densely written text.

Martin, S.J. and Green, D.R. (1995). Apoptosis and cancer: the failure of controls on cell death and cell survival. *Article Rev. Oncol. Hematol.*, 18: 137–153.

Morris, J.A. (1994). Information and clonal concepts in aging. *Med. Hypotheses*, 42: 89–92.

Rhoads, C.P. (1946). Nitrogen mustard in the treatment of neoplastic disease. *JAMA*, 131: 656–658.

Schoenlein, P.V. (1994). Role of gene amplification in drug resistance. In *Anticancer Drug Resistance: Adv. Mol. Clin. Res.* ed. L.J. Goldstein and R.F. Ozols, Kluwer Academic, New York.

Selivanova, G. and Wiman, K. (1995). p.53: a cell cycle regulator activated by DNA damage. *Adv. Cancer Res.*, 66: 143–180.

Tan, W.Y. and Gastardo, M.T.C. (1985). On the assessment of effects of environmental agents on cancer tumor development by a two-stage model of carcinogenesis. *Math. Biosci.*, 74: 143–155.

Tannock, I. and Hill, R.P. (1992). *The Basic Science of Oncology.* McGraw-Hill, New York. A very useful general introductory text to the cellular and molecular biology of cancer, with emphasis on phenomena that are felt to be of clinical relevance. Unlike many texts in this area the book is of manageable length.

Tisty, T.D., White, A., Livanos, E. *et al.* (1994). Genomic integrity and the genetics of cancer. *Cold Spring Harbor Symp. Quant. Biol.*, 59: 265–275.

Zubrod, C.G. (1979). Historic milestones in curative chemotherapy. *Sem. Oncol.*, 6: 490–505.

2

Tumour growth, stem cells and experimental chemotherapy

2.1 Introduction

Much of what has been learned concerning the properties of cancer cells has been developed from studies of a variety of cell lines that have been adapted for growth in tissue culture or in appropriate experimental animals. A variety of mammalian (chiefly rodent) and human cancer cell lines have been developed for this purpose. It has to be kept in mind that the properties of these highly selected experimental systems may differ from those that one might expect to find occurring in primary tumours in patients. Despite this caveat, it is apparent that many principles that have been learned from the experimental systems have been valuable in the understanding of human malignancy.

Any line of tumour cells that has adapted to growing in tissue culture or through serial transplantation in animals will have been subject to an extremely rigorous selection process. Normal (i.e. nonmalignant) fibroblasts in tissue culture will die out after they have undergone a number of sequential cell divisions (approximately 50). This appears to be the case no matter how carefully the culture conditions are established. This also appears to be true for many cancer cells in that there appears to be an upper limit to the number of sequential divisions they will undergo before becoming senescent and dying. Some tumour cells, however, become 'immortalized' and they will replicate indefinitely in the right type of environment. Recently, it has been suggested that an important step in the process whereby cells become immortal is related to the expression of the enzyme *telomerase*. Telomeres are repetitive sequences of DNA that occur at the ends of the chromosome. In normal somatic cells (but not germ cells or haematopoietic stem cells) the telomeres are progressively shortened after each cell division and this in some way signals the cell eventually to stop dividing. Telomerase prevents this progressive shortening of the telomere and this confers on the cell the capacity for continuous replication. Telomerase expression may occur at a late stage in the evolution of a tumour population either *in vivo* or *in vitro* and it may be these particular cellular phenotypes that are especially suitable for long-term culture. To date virtually every cell line that grows continuously in culture has been found positive when tested for telomerase activity. As telomerase could present a potential target for anticancer drugs it is currently a field of intensive investigation.

2.2   Growth of tumour cell populations

If cells growing in tissue culture or tumour cells that are inoculated into a host animal are regularly counted over time, one sees a progressive increase in cell number. If this increase is measured during the time before the tissue culture medium becomes exhausted, or before the transplanted tumour reaches some limiting size, it is noted that the tumour population will often grow at some nearly constant rate of doubling; that is, it grows at a rate proportional to its size at any instant of time. This steady proportional growth can be described as the circumstance when the logarithm of the increase in cell number per unit time is constant. Such growth can be described by the formula:

$$N(t) = N(0)e^{\lambda t} \qquad (2.1)$$

where $N(t)$ is the number of tumour cells present after an interval of time, t, which can be measured in any arbitrary unit of time (days, weeks, etc.). $N(0)$ is the number of tumour cells at the start of counting, e is the base of natural logarithms (2.71828 . . .)[†] and λ is the logarithm of growth. When plotted on a semilogarithmic graph, the increase in cell number follows a positive straight line, which results from a constant growth rate. This is described as logarithmic or exponential growth (Fig. 2.1). The actual slope of the exponential growth curve will be determined by the proportion of cells in the tumour that are dividing, their rate of division and the extent to which any spontaneous cell loss or death is occurring. In the simplest case where 100% of the cells are proliferating and there is no cell loss, the doubling time of the popula-

---

[†] e can be calculated from the term $y_n = y_0(1 + 1/n)^n$ where y_0 is the original value and y_n the value after n determinations. It represents the value by which an entity will increase at a compound interest rate when the interest is compounded, not yearly or daily, but at every instant of time.

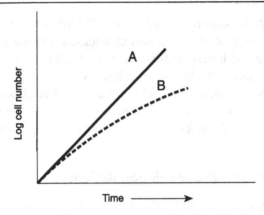

Fig. 2.1. Cell growth with time. A. Exponential or logarithmic growth. The tumour doubling time is constant (Equation 2.1). B. Gompertzian growth, showing progressive retardation in growth rate as tumour size increases. The tumour doubling time, which initially is nearly identical to that of the exponentially growing tumour, becomes progressively longer (Equation 2.2).

tion will be equal to the generation time of the component cells. Reductions in cell number can likewise be represented as a negative exponential with a cell population contracting at a constant rate of proportionality.

In practice, there are always deviations from a pure exponential growth function, with most clinical cancers deviating from their maximum potential growth by a considerable factor. The 'doubling time' of a tumour cell population is simply the time required for the population to increase its size by a factor of two. In clinical assessments of tumour growth it is usual to refer to the volume doubling time of the tumour as measured by sequential determinations of the volume of detectable clinical masses. Tumour volume and cell number can be related by the fact that a cubic centimetre of tumour tissue contains between 10^8 and 10^9 cells. A cubic centimetre of cells weighs approximately 1 gram, reflecting the fact that cells are composed mainly of water.

Many clinical tumours and some experimental 'solid' tumours can sometimes be described by growth functions in which the rate of growth declines with size. One popular function is the so called *Gompertz function* where the volume of the tumour instead of growing as a straight exponential undergoes progressive retardation as it approaches a limiting size. Mathematically it is described by

$$N(t) = N(0)\exp\left\{\frac{\lambda}{\beta}(1 - e^{-\beta t})\right\}$$ (2.2)

where λ and β are constants. (exp x denotes e raised to the power x, in this case the whole term $\{\lambda/\beta(1 - e^{-\beta t})\}$.) The log growth rate at time $t = 0$ is the same as the exponential (i.e. λ), but this declines as the tumour grows, eventually approaching zero. The Gompertz function was found to describe the growth of normal tissue systems that reach some naturally regulated size. Its ability to describe malignant systems, which by definition are not well regulated, is less convincing, though it is frequently used to describe malignant growth.

Basically the Gompertz function can simply be described as exponential growth that undergoes exponential retardation. The larger the size reached, the greater the degree of deceleration in the growth of the tumour. The growth of the tumour approaches but never reaches a plateau. Biologically, the Gompertzian shape of the growth function is possibly related to the fact that the growing tumour may exhaust its supply of nutrients as it increases in size or that there may be within the tumour cell population some negative feedback control process (Fig. 2.1).

In some models of tumour behaviour, critical importance is given to the Gompertzian nature of the growth function; however, from the perspective of somatic mutations, the precise form of the growth function does not change the final conclusions (Chapter 4). (This is because the number of mutations in a tumour is ultimately related to N, the tumour size, and total elapsed time rather than to any particular growth function.) Moreover, not infrequently clinical tumours appear to grow nearly exponentially during the time of clinical observation.

We referred to certain experimental tumours as being 'solid'; the term solid tumour is often used with respect to many types of clinical cancer. This is a somewhat misleading description as most neoplasms feel very solid to the touch, except those that grow in a widely dispersed form (e.g. leukaemia). In practical terms, solid tumour refers to those malignancies that as they grow generate their own blood supply (neovascularization or angiogenesis) on the periphery of the growing tumour mass. This is seen typically in epithelial malignancies (carcinomas) and mesenchymal tumours (sarcomas). Malignancies of the lymphoid and haematopoietic systems appear to generate less in the way of neovascularization than so-called solid tumours even when the lymphoid tumour has aggregated into a large mass. However, newer techniques are identifying what appear to be areas of neovascularization within lymphomatous and leukaemic masses, suggesting that the presence or absence of angiogenesis will not be sufficient to distinguish between lymphomas and solid tumours. Haematological malignancies are generally described as simply lymphomas/leukaemias or, sometimes, liquid tumours.

2.3   Cell renewal systems

In a typical transplantable mouse leukaemia, nearly all of the cells constituting the leukaemic tissue appear as morphologically undifferentiated malignant cells and virtually all of them are capable of indefinite cell replication. That is, each single cell constituting the leukaemia will divide to form two daughter cells, each of which will divide to form two more daughter cells, etc. In this respect, the experimental leukaemia resembles a population of bacteria where each bacterium divides to form two virtually identical bacteria, and these undergo further divisions. In these systems, a single leukaemic cell or single bacterium can, in theory, reproduce itself indefinitely.

This property is in contrast to what is observed for the vast majority of normally functioning cells in an organism. Most of the cells that make up an animal are highly differentiated cells that have developed specialized biochemical and morphological features and that display little or no capacity for cell division. Moreover the life span of many of these cells appears limited and they are replaced by newer cells that are produced as a consequence of division of less differentiated cells. These differentiated cells, even if they can carry out a few rounds of cell replication, would fail to produce a countable colony in a viability assay and would be considered in an operational sense as 'dead'. That is, they are effectively sterile and cannot contribute to the continued growth of the population.

With some tissues, virtually no cell turnover takes place once embryonic and early childhood growth is complete (e.g. the neurons of the central nervous system). However, there are a number of cell systems in the body, such as the digestive tract and the haematopoietic system, where there is continuous production of new cells. The new cells acquire progressively more specialized function and finally become senescent and undergo dissolution. Tissues with such a continuous rate of cell turnover are generally described as *cell renewal* systems; among the best studied of these, and perhaps of particular relevance to many types of malignancy, is the haematopoietic system.

2.4 The spleen colony assay and the concept of renewal probability

It had long been suspected that in a tissue such as the bone marrow the vast majority of the morphologically distinguishable cells must have been derived from more primitive cells with a greater replicative potential. These cells were felt to be analogous to the cells present in the developing embryo in so far as they had a capacity to undergo cell division and to give rise to a lineage of differentiated cells. They were referred to as *stem cells* because of their progenitor function within the tissue system.

In the early 1960s, James Till and Ernest McCulloch in Toronto developed a quantitative *in vivo* assay system for measuring the stem cell component of mouse bone marrow (Till, McCulloch and Simonovitch, 1964). The method described is known as the mouse spleen colony assay. In this assay, bone marrow cells are removed from one of the long bones of a normal mouse and then a known number of these cells are injected into a second mouse that has received a high dose of total body irradiation. The radiation is used to suppress all endogenous haematopoiesis (Fig. 2.2). After 7 days the mice are killed and their spleens removed. A large number of visible nodules are detected in the spleen and it has been shown that each nodule represents a colony of normal haematopoietic cells derived from a single progenitor cell. This assay thus permits the investigator to estimate the frequency of colony-forming cells (or stem cells) per total number of nucleated marrow cells. The results suggested that there is one colony-forming cell per 5000 or more nucleated cells.

The individual colonies in the spleen can then be removed and injected into a second recipient mouse. The number of secondary colonies seen can then be used to measure the capacity of the original bone marrow cells to undergo the production of new stem cells (*self-renewal*). From these studies, Till and McCulloch were able to build up a mathematical model of the behaviour of the marrow cells with respect to their capacity to undergo replication. The investigators concluded that whether or not an individual stem cell divided to form two new stem

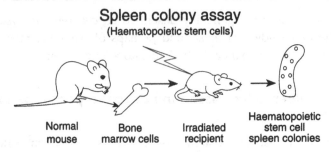

Spleen colony assay
(Haematopoietic stem cells)

| Normal
mouse | Bone
marrow cells | Irradiated
recipient | Haematopoietic
stem cell
spleen colonies |

Fig. 2.2. Technique for assaying the number of bone marrow stem cells. A normal mouse is killed and a cell suspension is made from the marrow of the mouse's thigh bone. A known number of nucleated marrow cells are injected intravenously into a second mouse that is of the same strain as the first. The second mouse has been heavily irradiated to suppress all endogenous haematopoietic growth, permitting the injected marrow cells to proliferate. After 7 days the spleen is removed from the recipient mouse and a number of discrete nodules can be observed in the spleen. These are counted and the results from a large number of individual mice can be pooled. The relationship between the number of spleen nodules and the number of injected marrow cells can be established. By using techniques such as chromosome marking, each nodule can be shown to be a clonal colony of haematopoietic cells. In separate experiments, the fraction of injected marrow cells that land in the spleen can be estimated. Individual colonies can be removed from the spleen, made into a suspension and then injected into a third mouse. This will measure the capacity of the colony-forming cells to form new colonies (self-renewal).

cells was a random event that would occur with a certain probability, P (the renewal probability). The reverse probability of the stem cell division giving rise to two differentiated cells was therefore $1 - P$ (Fig. 2.3).

For any cell system that is increasing its numbers over time, it is apparent that cell birth (P) must be greater than cell deaths or differentiation ($1 - P$). In regenerating bone marrow, the renewal probability was found to be approximately 0.53, but when the marrow had regenerated to its original physiological level the renewal probability appears to fall to close to 0.5. If the renewal probability is less than 0.5, then the population will progressively diminish until it is extinguished.

Since the renewal probability of the normal haematopoietic system lies close to 0.5 and the choice of renewal is random, there is always the probability of more deaths than births and, hence, the whole population becoming extinct. It is possible to calculate the probability, P_{ext}, that a

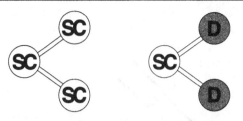

Renewal probability = P.   Differentiation probability = 1 - P

Fig. 2.3. Schematic representations of the renewal probability concept for haematopoietic stem cells. At each division the cell has a certain probability, P, to give rise to two new stem cells, or to give rise to two differentiated cells (which by definition lose stem cell capacity) with probability 1 − P. The overall probability of self-renewal for the entire population of stem cells can be estimated, but whether any individual cell undergoes self-renewal is random.

single stem cell line will die out. The probability that two cells will become extinct, assuming cells to behave independently, is $(P_{ext})^2$. Therefore, P_{ext} is equal to the probability that no stem cells are produced at the first division, $1 - P$, plus the probability that two stem cells are produced, P, multiplied by the probability that both cells will go extinct $(P_{ext})^2$:

$$P_{ext} = 1 - P + (P_{ext})^2 \times P.$$

Solving this equation yields

$$P_{ext} = \frac{1 - P}{P} \tag{2.3}$$

for $P > 0.5$; for $P \leq 0.5$, $P_{ext} = 1$. The probability of extinction of N independent stem cells is:

$$(P_{ext})^N = \left(\frac{1 - P}{P}\right)^N$$

The closer P lies to 0.5 and the smaller the value for N, then the greater the likelihood of extinction. If $P = 0.5$ the system will eventually become extinct with 100% probability, no matter how large the population (i.e. $[(1 - 0.5)/0.5] = 1$). If N is large, however, the probability of extinction occurring rapidly will be very small (Fig. 2.4).

This relationship holds true for a broad range of phenomena and is not simply confined to dividing cells. It is also applied to populations of

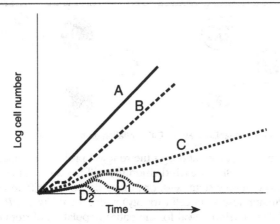

Fig. 2.4. Four computer-generated growth curves of a tumour population in which the renewal probability P is varied. Curve A represents a renewal of probability 1, in which there is no cell loss and the system grows as a pure exponential with its doubling time equal to its generation time. B displays a renewal probability of 0.8. The system grows slightly slower than A, and there is slight irregularity of growth when the population is small. C has a renewal probability of 0.58. Growth shows further slowing and there is a longer period of irregularity at low cell numbers. D, D_1 and D_2 show renewal probabilities of 0.52. The three simulations shown all become extinct within a relatively short time of growth commencement. It would take a large number of trials (10 or more) before a population, by chance, would reach a size sufficient to make extinction highly unlikely.

animals and also for chain reactions involving subatomic particles. The renewal probability theorem is part of a general field of mathematics called branching processes or, more specifically, birth/death processes.

The concept of renewal probability has proved to be very useful in describing the behaviour of the normal haematopoietic system and, as it turns out, for studying the behaviour of cancer cell populations as well. The Till and McCulloch model of a cell renewal system postulates that the component cells are divided into three main compartments (Fig. 2.5) The first compartment is made up of the stem cells which have the properties of both extensive proliferation and self-renewal. The operative word here is extensive because, as mentioned above, normal cells probably lack the capacity to replicate indefinitely. In experiments where bone marrow colony-forming cells were serially transplanted from one mouse to another, the colony-forming efficiency eventually starts to decline. However, the proliferation potential of the marrow

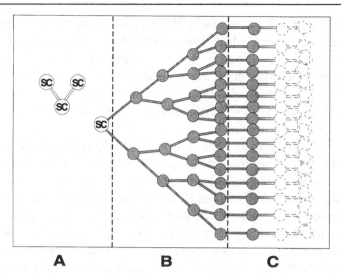

Fig. 2.5. Three-compartment model for a cell-renewal system such as the haematopoietic system or a malignant neoplasm. A. The stem cell compartment where cells can either undergo self-renewal or commence differentiation. B. The differentiation or *transitional* cell compartment. These cells undergo morphological and functional changes (which will generally be highly abnormal in tumours) and a variable number of divisions until they finally lose proliferative capacity. The number of divisions is sometimes referred to as the clonal expansion number. C. A compartment composed of fully differentiated terminal or end cells. In a normal cell system, they carry out the physiological function of the tissue from which they are derived. They will have a variable life span, which, depending on the tissue of origin, can range from a few days to many years. The larger the clonal expansion number and the longer the half life of the end cells, then the smaller the proportion of actual stem cells that will be present.

stem cells is still very great and is sufficient to maintain it over a normal lifetime. In the mouse, a single colony-forming cell can reconstitute the marrow of a recipient mouse in which there is a congenital deficiency of marrow stem cell function.

The second compartment of the renewal system is made up of cells that have retained a limited capacity for proliferation and that also at the same time undergo progressive differentiation, acquiring the properties of a fully mature cell. Under the influence of a series of specific growth factors, the differentiating cell begins producing new proteins and altering its morphological appearance. At the end of six to ten sequential divisions, there will be terminally differentiated cells such as erythrocytes or granulocytes, which have ceased division permanently. The number of divisions carried out by these differentiating cells is usually referred to as the clonal expansion number. During the process of clonal expansion, the progeny of a single stem cell may give rise to a thousand or more fully differentiated cells depending on the actual value for the clonal expansion number.

The third compartment is made up of terminally differentiated or end cells, which no longer have the capacity to undergo cell division. They have a finite life span ranging from a few days to 3 to 4 months, but they eventually become senescent, undergo apoptosis and are removed. The maintenance of the end-cell compartment requires a continuous input from the less-differentiated cells. If the stem cell compartment is suddenly depleted (by exposure to radiation or a cytotoxic agent), the effects will be first observed in the cells with the shortest life span and quickest turnover (granulocytes, platelets) and will be much less apparent with the long-lived cells such as erythrocytes.

We can summarize by saying a stem cell has several properties: (a), it has a capacity for extensive proliferation and self-renewal, (b) it is able to give rise to an expanding clone of differentiating cells and (c) it responds to a series of physiological growth signals for both commencing and ceasing cell division.

2.5   A stem cell model for cancer

A number of different lines of evidence suggests that the cellular make-up of tumours, particularly primary tumours in animals and humans, has many similarities to the cellular organization of cell renewal systems such as the bone marrow. In many clinical tumours there is often very significant morphological evidence of cellular differentiation occurring with abnormal but still recognizable, differentiated cells present. These partially differentiated cells may make up the great bulk of cells in the tumour and provide one of the important clues as to the tissue and cell of origin of the malignant cells. In certain malignant disorders of the haematopoietic system, such as polycythemia vera and chronic myelogenous leukaemia, the terminally differentiated cells are still able to carry out important physiological functions. In polycythemia for example, virtually all of the erythrocytes present in the patient will be derived from a malignant clone but nonetheless are capable of oxygen and carbon dioxide transport.

In many malignancies, morphological differentiation may not be readily apparent but tests of cell viability will reveal that only a small proportion of the cancer cells are capable of division and that an even smaller number actually undergoing self-renewal. (See review by MacKillop et al., 1983). As was pointed out by Bush and Hill (1975), most clinical cancers would not be curable by the usual doses of radiation employed therapeutically if it were the case that all of the component cells of the tumour had stem cell function. Their conclusion was based in part on the observation that experimental tumours, which are nearly 100% stem cells, require a much larger dose of radiation to cure than a clinical tumour of equivalent volume. (Animal and human cancer cells are roughly equivalent in their radiosensitivity.) A 1 gram (10^9 cells) clinical tumour might contain a thousand times fewer stem cells than an experimental tumour and, therefore, effectively be one thousand times 'smaller'. It could be inferred that with some malignancies as few as 1 cell per 10^5 morphologically abnormal cells might actually be a true self-renewing stem cell. This implies that the effective biological size of the tumour may be only approximately related to its volume and the number of countable cells present in that volume.

The stem cell model of clinical cancer has a number of important implications for cancer biology as well as for devising therapeutic strategies. Firstly, the number of actual tumour stem cells (often referred to as *clonogenic cells*) that need to be killed or sterilized will generally only be a small fraction of the total number of cells present in the tumour. This makes the job of the radiation therapist easier but, as will be seen below, not necessarily that of the chemotherapist.

Another important implication of the stem cell model of cancer relates to the fact that there will be a considerable difference between the potential doubling time of the tumour (T_{pot}) and the actual doubling time of the entire neoplastic population.

Since a proportion, P, of divisions produce 2 stem cells ($2 \times P$) while a proportion ($1 - P$) produces none ($1 - P \times 0$), the relationship between the generation time of the component tumour stem cells and the overall doubling time of the tumour can be derived from the renewal probability. In a stable renewal system, the proportional increase in the overall size of the population is ($2P$) at every division. Thus after n divisions the proportional increase is ($2P)^n$, so that the value of n for which this increase is twofold represents the doubling time, measured in multiples of the generation time. Therefore, we have $(2P)^n = 2$, so that

$$n = \left[1 + \frac{\log 2}{\log 2P}\right] - 1$$

and the doubling time of the tumour is given by

$$T_{\text{doub}} = n \times T_{\text{Div}} = \left[1 + \frac{\log 2}{\log 2P}\right]^{-1} \times T_{\text{Div}} \qquad (2.4)$$

where T_{Div} is the generation time of the stem cells. For example, if the generation time is 24 hours (1 day) and the renewal probability is 0.52, then the overall doubling time will be 17.7 days. If the renewal probability is 0.51 and the generation time is 48 hours then the doubling time will be 70 days for the system.

Over the long term, the doubling time of the tumour will be determined by the generation time and renewal probability of the stem cells. This will be true even if the differentiated cells have very short generation times. They will contribute to the growth rate of the tumour during the earliest phase of growth only. Once the differentiated cells cease dividing, the system will come to an equilibrium with only the growth of the stem cells determining the overall growth rate. (This will be discussed again in Chapter 6. A rigorous proof of this theorem would require a detailed discussion of branching process theory.)

Note that it is possible to have a very long doubling time for a tumour system and still have the generation times of the component stem cells very short. Many human tumours have doubling times in the range 50–100 days. As we have seen, however, this does *not* mean that the generation times of the tumour stem cells need be anything like as long.

Most human cancer cells that can be grown in tissue culture have generation times in the order of 24–48 hours. In human tumour stem cell assays, detectable colonies can be seen in less than 14 days. If the generation times of the stem cells were the same as the clinical doubling time of the tumour, it would take many weeks to produce a countable colony.

If the renewal probability is exactly 0.5, then the doubling time of the system is infinite. However, when the renewal probability lies close to 1 then the doubling time is almost equal to the generation time, a circumstance seen in transplantable leukaemias. Very rapidly growing human tumours, say with a generation time of 24 hours and a renewal probability of 0.65, would display a doubling time of about 2.5 days. This is close to the maximum growth rate that is observed in human malignancy and suggests some upper bound on the renewal probability that primary human tumour stem cells are likely to display.

Depending on the average half life of the nondividing end cells in the tumour, measurable fluctuations in tumour size following therapy may appear to be very fast or slow. Tumours with a rapid turnover of cells, such as certain lymphomas and acute leukaemias, may show a sudden and steep drop in cell numbers even if the log kill value is relatively small. In these circumstances, it will be the time elapsed before the tumour again reaches its pretreatment size that will be the true measure of therapeutic effect.

If a tumour is already undergoing a significant degree of differentiation, this provides an important rationale for increasing the likelihood of differentiation by treating the tumour with pharmacological doses of some type of differentiation inducer. This will have the effect of reducing the value of the renewal probability and, concomitantly, increase the value of $1 - P$, the differentiation probability. This strategy is employed in certain malignancies, and sometimes with considerable effect. Promyelocytic leukaemia responds to high doses of analogues of retinoic acid, and useful responses can be obtained in prostate and breast cancer by employing the appropriate hormonal agent, which basically operates to increase the degree of cellular differentiation and apoptosis in these hormonally responsive tumours.

2.6 Chemotherapy of experimental leukaemia

Many of our present concepts of cancer chemotherapy have been derived from a series of papers written in the 1960s by Howard Skipper, Frank Schabel and colleagues at the Southern Research Institute in Alabama (Skipper, Schabel and Wilcox, 1964). These workers sought to put the chemotherapy of cancer on a firm quantitative basis. Their work has become such an accepted background to the field of cancer chemotherapy that it is somewhat difficult to convey the sense of profound enlightenment that accompanied the initial appearance of their studies.

One of the major experimental models that Skipper and Schabel relied upon was the transplantable L1210 leukaemia in mice. This system consists of a line of mouse lymphatic leukaemia (or lymphoma) cells that are maintained by transplantation from one highly inbred mouse to another. These mice are virtually genetically identical and a spontaneous malignancy developing in one of them can be transplanted to another mouse of the same strain without the tumour cells undergoing immunological rejection. If this process is carried on through a large number of transplant generations, then the tumour cells become very homogeneous and quite predictable in terms of their behaviour. This makes it possible to inoculate large numbers of mice of the same age with the same number of leukaemia cells and observe a very similar clinical course in each individual animal. The experimental conditions are thus highly reproducible and sufficient numbers of individual animals can be obtained for a particular experimental endpoint. There are obviously biological differences between these experimental tumour systems and the spontaneous malignancies that arise in human beings, but there appear to be sufficient similarities to the clinical disease that many of the lessons learned from studying the transplanted leukaemias can be applied clinically.

From Skipper's studies, a number of very important principles relating to cancer chemotherapy and cancer biology were established.

Principle I Animals will die when their total body burden of malignant cells reaches some critical number, which is very similar for animals of similar size

If a small number of leukaemic cells (say between 100 and 1000) are inoculated into a recipient animal then these will, after a short delay, grow exponentially with time until they reach a value of approximately one billion (10^9) cells. At this point, the host animal becomes ill and will generally die within a few hours. The larger the size of the initial inoculum then, generally, the shorter the lag period before the tumour population begins to grow; in addition, there is less variation in time between the inoculation and the animal's death.

This is the so-called *lethal number* of cancer cells that is required to kill a host animal. The population of malignant cells has to reach a certain general range of numbers before it can have a sufficient impact on the homeostatic processes going on within the host to result in the organism's death. This concept of a lethal number can also be applied to the circumstances involving microbial infection, but it is less commonly used when discussing the chemotherapy of infectious diseases.

However, the concept of lethal number has proved to be a very valuable one in experimental and clinical oncology (Fig. 2.6). The lethal number of cancer cells for an organism bears a direct relationship to the size of the animal. For a mouse, the lethal number is approximately 10^9 cells, for a rat 10^{10} and for a human being 10^{12}. This is only approximate, of course, and the actual number will depend on the location of the tumour and whether it is widespread (as in leukaemia). For a disseminated malignancy like leukaemia, the lethal number in a patient is close to 10^{12}, whereas for a brain tumour it would be closer to 10^{11}.

Principle 2 A single viable leukaemic cell is sufficient to produce the clinical disease and kill the animal

By using special techniques to inject a single viable cell into the recipient animal, Skipper concluded that a single surviving leukaemic cell is sufficient to reconstitute the disease. Therefore, curative chemotherapy has to be capable of destroying all of the viable leukaemic cells in the animal and within tolerable limits of toxicity.

Single malignant cells can be injected into an animal by using a micromanipulator, which is basically a tiny pipette that under micro-

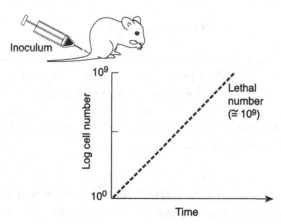

Fig. 2.6. Exponential growth of mouse leukaemia following injection of approximately one cell. The number of malignant cells grow with a constant doubling time (8–10 hours) until they reach approximately 10^9 cells. This constitutes a lethal burden of malignant cells for the animal, which will die within a short time of the lethal number being reached.

scopic control can be used to withdraw a single cell from a cell suspension. The single cell is then injected into a recipient animal; while a proportion of the cells acquired in this way may be damaged and non-viable, some will survive the procedure and the technique can allow the influence of a single cell when injected to be assessed.

As this method is technically difficult, another approach is to employ the principle of limiting dilution. In this technique, the number of leukaemic cells in a known volume of fluid is counted. The volume of fluid is then serially diluted until it is estimated that there is, on average, one cell per culture tube. Obviously, identical replicate samples processed in the same way will not all have one remaining cell per culture, or whatever the average is, but will display a distribution with some counts greater than the mean and some less. The appropriate distribution in such situations is the Poisson distribution. (The Poisson distribution is a good approximation of the binomial distribution where the probability of a particular event occurring is very low but the number of opportunities for the events to happen is large.) The derivation of this distribution is not an appropriate topic here but we will give its mathematical description as we will use it considerably later.

If X is the number of cells actually present in the culture and μ is the average number expected, then the probability that X will be equal to some integer value, x say, is $P\{X = x\}$ and is given by

$$P\{X = x\} = \frac{\mu^x e^{-\mu}}{x!}. \tag{2.5}$$

The most important property of the distribution for our purposes is that the probability of no cells, $P\{X = 0\}$, is equal to $e^{-\mu}$ (since $0! = 1$).

It transpires that when the dilution has been carried to the point where there is an average of one cell per tube the actual distribution will show approximately 1/3 of the tubes having zero cells, 1/3 will have 1 and 1/3 will have 2 or more.

Principle 3   The increase in survival time seen in treated animals is directly related to the magnitude of the log kill produced by treatment

If the leukaemic animals are treated at a point well before the number of cancer cells approaches the lethal number, then measurements can be made of the average prolongation of life that is obtained with a particular dose of drug. It is assumed that the killing of the cells by the drug happens nearly instantaneously, and the surviving leukaemic cell population then begins to grow back at its previous rate. From these experiments it is possible to extrapolate the growth of the tumour back in time to calculate the proportion of malignant cells that were killed at the time of drug exposure (Fig. 2.7).

Principle 4 A given dose of a chemotherapeutic agent would always kill about the same proportion or fraction of the leukaemic cells present in the animal

The absolute number of leukaemic cells killed by a course of therapy will vary depending upon whether there was a larger or lesser number of malignant cells present when the treatment was applied. If the dose of

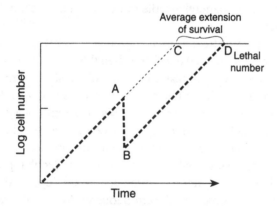

Fig. 2.7. Log kill effect on exponentially growing mouse leukaemia. Treatment is given at point A when there is a known burden of leukaemic cells present. This reduces the tumour burden to the level at point B. There are two groups of animals: those treated and the control group, which are untreated. The untreated animals reach the lethal burden of tumour cells at point C. The treated animals survive longer to point D. A line parallel to AC is drawn from D. A line parallel to the y axis is dropped from A. This intersects the line from C at point B. Point B represents the nadir of the fall in leukaemic cell numbers after treatment. The log kill of the treatment can be read off the y axis. The average extension of life in the treated animals is represented by CD, which can be seen to be directly related to AB (the log kill). With bigger or more doses of drug the nadir reached will be lower and survival longer. If the entire leukaemic population is destroyed then the animals will be cured ('indefinite' survival).

the particular drug was increased then it would be observed that a greater fraction of the leukaemic cells were killed and, likewise, if the dose was decreased there would be a smaller fraction. In other words, the log kill of the chemotherapeutic agent is related to the dose of drug and not to the absolute number of leukaemic cells present.

We can note in passing that the question of log kill or mean cell survival probability can be expressed mathematically in the same way as was used to describe the cell renewal probability for the birth/death process. In the cell renewal systems where the term P referred to the renewal probability and $1 - P$ to the probability of differentiation, we can consider processes such as differentiation as being functionally equivalent to being killed. That is, the cell permanently loses the capacity for proliferation. Moreover, it can be stated more generally that, in the renewal probability equation, the term $1 - P$ simply refers to the probability of cell loss, death or differentiation, or indeed to any process that renders the cell permanently sterile or no longer a functional part of the cellular system.

If under the impact of treatment, the average renewal probability of an L1210 leukaemia falls from 0.8 to 0.008 then this would mean that the total leukaemic stem cell population would diminish in terms of its viability by three logs. Concomitantly, the process of cell loss, or death, is increased by the same amount. This apparent coincidence in terms of the mathematical relationships between self-renewal and chemotherapy killing effects may be more than coincidental, as will be discussed in a later chapter when some of the molecular processes that are initiated during chemotherapeutic action are described.

It used to be sometimes said (erroneously) that since numbers expressed as a logarithm never assume the value of 0 then the log kill effect of chemotherapy could never actually cure an animal. That is, a three log kill directed against a tumour population of 10^2 would result in 1/10th of a cell surviving per animal, obviously an impossibility. The logic is flawed here because when we use the term log kill we are referring to the average probability of cell survival. The three log kill effect would mean that there would be, on average, 90% of a group of animals cured and 10% with at least one surviving cell. A dose of drug sufficient to produce a four log kill against a burden of 10^2 cells would mean that animal had a 99% chance of cure (but there would be the one animal per 100 treated that would survive by chance alone).

Principle 5   As a single surviving leukaemic cell might be sufficient to cause disease relapse, treatment has to be extended well past the point of clinical remission

The potential for a single cell to initiate relapse means carrying on with the treatment for several courses past the time where all clinical signs have disappeared. In these transplanted leukaemias, there appears to be little or no immune response directed against the malignant cells and providing the surviving cell is capable of stem cell function then one cell will be sufficient (in theory) to regrow and cause clinical leukaemia. This is a problem with transplanted leukaemias in particular, because it would appear that with these cell lines most of the component cells function as stem cells with a high renewal probability. The renewal probability is almost certainly not 1, but probably lies between 0.6 and 0.8. With renewal probabilities that high, then the doubling time of the tumour will only be slightly greater than that of the generation time of the component cells, and a single surviving cell would have a significant probability of reconstituting the disease. For example, if the renewal probability P is 0.8 then the extinction probability of a population of 10 stem cells P_{ext} is 1×10^{-6}; for P 0.6, P_{ext} is 0.02. In contrast, if we were dealing with populations of malignant stem cells whose renewal probabilities are 0.51 then the extinction probability remains high with $P_{ext} = 0.67$. In these instances, it may only be necessary to reduce the surviving stem cell population to a relatively small number (for example between 1 and 25) for there still to be a significant probability of the residual tumour dying out.

Principle 6   There is a relationship between tumour burden at the time of therapy initiation and the likelihood of cure

It was recognized that a large number of tumour cells would require more courses of treatment to achieve cure than a smaller number, but it was repeatedly noted in the L1210 leukaemia that if the tumour burden was about 10^6 at the time treatment was commenced a few animals would be cured. If the tumour burden was $< 10^5$, then nearly 100% cures were observed. If the tumour burden was very large, 10^8 or greater, then the cure rate was virtually zero. This was true no matter how many courses of treatment were applied. It was observed during the course of treatment that after initial very substantial regression of the leukaemic cell population regrowth could occur and might be unaffected by applications of treatment that had been initially successful in causing tumour response.

When the leukaemic cells from animals that died of recurrent disease were harvested and inoculated in small numbers into new recipient animals, it was found that these selected leukaemic populations were essentially invulnerable to the doses of chemotherapy that had previously been effective in curing the leukaemia in the initial animals. This suggested that whatever was responsible for the resistance of the leukaemia was something that resided primarily at the level of the individual cell.

It was not a general resistance phenomenon because the use of a different type of chemotherapeutic agent would result in very substantial tumour regression and would cure the animals if the tumour population was relatively low at the time therapy was commenced. Moreover, there were no obvious gross differences in the behaviour of the resistant tumour cells compared with the original sensitive cell population. Morphologically, the tumour cells appeared identical, and their growth rate was virtually the same. This appeared to represent a classical example of acquired chemotherapeutic resistance that bore many similarities to the phenomenon that was regularly being encountered in the clinical chemotherapy of leukaemia and other malignancies.

Principle 7 The size and frequency of drug dose are critical variables in determining cure

It is perhaps self-evident that the dose level, frequency of dosing and total number of doses would clearly influence whether or not the animals would be cured, even if their tumours were inherently very sensitive to the chemotherapy. If the size of dose was too small and the interval was too long between doses, then there would be, in effect, a negative net log kill with the tumour population 'gaining' on the therapy. Likewise, if the treatment was stopped before eradication of all viable cells, then treatment failure would result. In a very rapidly growing neoplasm such as the L1210 leukaemia, such timing factors were of critical importance. In treating tumours *in vivo* (experimental or clinical) the upper limits of dose are set by the toxicity effects in normal tissues. In *in vitro* experiments, concentrations of drugs can be increased to any arbitrary level, but in clinical chemotherapy a 5% treatment-associated mortality ordinarily would be considered as close to the limit of acceptable toxicity. (This is for circumstances where a significant cure rate is possible. It would be unacceptable in palliative situations.)

Subsequently, in 1984, Hryniuk and Bush developed the concept of *dose intensity* in which the ratio of drug dose and drug timing was introduced. (Chapter 7).

Principle 8   Two or more agents given concurrently or sequentially will produce cures when single agents have failed

The amount of drug given to an animal is limited by the toxicity of the agent to the whole animal. In a petri dish, there is no problem to the dish. Skipper and Schabel were able to demonstrate consistently the greatly enhanced curative potential of combination chemotherapy compared with single agents (Skipper *et al.*, 1964). This could be seen if the multiple agents were given concurrently or if one agent was given first to the point of maximal net log kill and then treatment was switched to the second (the 'treat to nadir and switch' strategy).

The principle of combination chemotherapy has emerged as perhaps the single most important stratagem that can be brought to bear in cancer chemotherapy. Clinical tests of combination chemotherapy were being started at this time, but the experimental work provided a powerful rationale for this approach and suggested that cellular drug resistance was the problem that the multiple drug therapy was overcoming.

The ability to monitor the tumour burden in the treated animals made it possible to fine tune the treatments according to these principles. It is very much harder (or often impossible) to do these kinds of estimate in clinical situations.

2.7   The cell cycle

We have already made a brief reference to the cell cycle, which is associated with cell division. The cell cycle (generation cycle, division cycle) refers to the series of events that occur in every somatic cell each time it divides. An analogous process occurs in the germ cells as they divide, but in this case there is a step that involves halving of the chromosome number in each cell (meiosis), which is in contrast to the doubling of the number of chromosomes that occurs in the somatic cells.

The cell cycle represents a sequence of morphological and molecular events that occurs from one cellular mitosis to the next (Fig. 2.8). Early studies in the 1950s established the main subdivisions of the events of the cell cycle. The most easily distinguishable event is the formation of the mitotic apparatus in the cell immediately prior to the actual fission of the cell into two progeny. At this point, each pair of chromosomes separates with a set of 23 pairs of chromosomes moving to the opposite poles of the cell prior to actual cell division.

The early cytologists described the stages in the movement of the chromosomes as prophase, anaphase, metaphase and telophase. After cell division, there was a long period of time when there did not appear to be much occurring within the cell (except that cell volume steadily increased; otherwise, of course, the cell would halve its size each time it divided) and then the mitotic apparatus would become visible again and once more division would occur. The long 'quiet' period between mitoses was designated as *interphase*. In the 1950s Howard and Pelc utilizing radiolabelled thymidine were able to demonstrate that DNA synthesis commenced several hours after mitosis and then ceased a few hours prior to the next mitosis (Howard and Pelc, 1953). This period was called the DNA synthetic phase or S. The two intervals between M and S and S and M were known, respectively, as the first and second postmitotic gaps, shortened to G_1 and G_2. The 'gap' referred to the fact

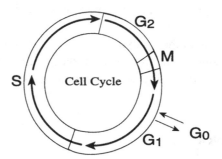

Fig. 2.8. The major phases of the cell cycle. At mitosis (M) the cell divides to form daughter cells. The cell may pass on through the next phase (G_1) to commence duplication of the DNA content at S, it may enter a physiological quiescent stage (G_0) or it may commence both differentiation and DNA synthesis. In normal cell systems a very complex and finely balanced control system operates to regulate the movement through each point in the cell cycle. (See text.)

that almost nothing was known about what was occurring during these intervals. In a typical cell in culture, the time elapsed from mitosis to mitosis was some 24 to 48 hours in human cells and 8 to 12 hours in mouse cells. DNA synthesis occupied about 25 to 50% of the total cell cycle time and M mitosis approximately 1 hour. (DNA synthesis occurs at many points simultaneously along the DNA molecule. If this did not happen it has been estimated that it would take several months for the DNA in a chromosome to replicate itself.)

Since the early 1960s, much information has been acquired concerning the events of the cell cycle and their relation to the malignant state. It is now known that the G_1 phase involves a number of crucial steps in which the cell makes decisions regarding whether it stops dividing, enters a differentiation pathway, repairs damage to its DNA, initiates apoptosis or proceeds to the next round of DNA synthesis. A number of investigators have long suspected that the control processes in the cell cycle were fundamental to the nature of malignancy. Recent studies have abundantly confirmed this, indicating that many of the key signal pathways regulated by both the oncogenes and tumour suppressor genes operate by controlling the sequence of events in the cell cycle.

2.8   The kinetic classification of chemotherapeutic agents

Shortly after Skipper and colleagues published their seminal work on experimental leukaemia, Bruce and co-workers in Toronto reported studies on the differential effects of chemotherapy on normal versus malignant cells (Bruce, Meaker and Valeriote, 1966). These workers utilized the bone marrow colony-forming assay of Till and McCulloch to quantify the effect of chemotherapy on a normal cell system, while employing a similar type of assay for mouse lymphoma cells.

In their technique, a transplanted mouse lymphoma line (AKR) was used (similar in many respects to the mouse L1210 leukaemia). A known number of lymphoma cells was injected intravenously into mice and the number of lymphoma nodules that developed in the spleen was counted after 7 days (Fig. 2.9). It was not necessary to radiate the animals to suppress normal haematopoiesis under these conditions. Exactly as in the bone marrow assay, the number of cells capable of producing colonies could be enumerated. With the transplanted lymphoma cells, a very high proportion of the cells was capable of producing colonies, which were in turn found to contain a further high proportion of sec-

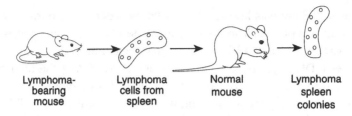

Lymphoma-   Lymphoma   Normal   Lymphoma
bearing   cells from   mouse   spleen
mouse   spleen   colonies

Fig. 2.9. The lymphoma colony-forming cell assay. A mouse that has been injected with lymphoma cells is killed when the lymphoma is far advanced. The spleen, which is now heavily infiltrated with lymphoma cells, is made into a suspension and a known number of spleen cells (which will be mainly lymphoma) is injected into a normal mouse. After 7 days the injected animals are killed and lymphoma colonies in the spleen can be counted in the same way as bone marrow spleen colonies. It is not necessary to irradiate the mice as the lymphoma cells will grow in normal splenic tissue.

ondary colony-forming cells. That is, the renewal probability of the transplanted lymphoma cells was very high, and similar to that which had been observed for the L1210 leukaemia.

This high proportion of colony-forming cells in the tumour population was in marked contrast to what was observed (Bruce and van der Gaag, 1963) when the colony-forming efficiency of the spontaneous mouse AKR lymphoma was evaluated. Mice of the AKR strain will come down with a spontaneous lymphoma at approximately 6 months of age. The biology of this tumour is probably closer to the biology of spontaneous malignancies in humans than to a transplanted tumour cell population. In the spontaneous AKR lymphoma, it was noted that there was a considerable variation from animal to animal in the proportion of colony-forming cells per total number of malignant cells. Individual animals with what appeared to be tumours at an identical stage showed very significant variability in the capacity of their tumour cells to generate spleen colonies. The numbers ranged from 1 colony-forming cell per 10^2 morphologically malignant cells to as low as 1 colony-forming cell per 10^5 malignant cells. The colony-forming efficiency of this very homogeneous-appearing spontaneous tumour varied over a range of three orders of magnitude. However, after sublines of this tumour had been transplanted over many generations, the variability from animal to animal disappeared, resulting in a tumour cell population with a very high colony-forming efficiency.

In Bruce's experiments (Bruce *et al.*, 1966), normal animals and animals with advanced transplanted AKR lymphoma were given graded doses of a number of antineoplastic agents. For each dose level the number of surviving haematopoietic colony-forming cells and of surviving lymphoma colony-forming cells were estimated and the dose response curves for both types of cell were then plotted. Utilizing a variety of antineoplastic agents, Bruce found that there appeared to be three types of dose response curve obtained. In each instance, the dose response curves of the normal and malignant cells were of similar shape, but in two categories a significant quantitative difference between the effect on the normal versus the malignant cell population was noted. The categories of dose response were designated as classes I, II and III (Fig. 2.10).

Class I agents included ionizing radiation and the drug nitrogen mustard, which produced a linear dose response relationship. In this circumstance the decline in cell viability of the normal versus malignant cells was identical. The class II group of agents produced a sigmoid dose response curve with an initial rapid falling off in viability followed by a plateau with increasing dose. There was, however, a significant quantitative difference in the effect of the drugs on the malignant versus the normal cell population, with the latter being much less sensitive to the cytotoxic effect. The drugs in this category included agents such as methotrexate, cytosine arabinoside (ara-C), vincristine and high-dose tritiated thymidine.

The last category of dose response effect (class III) was seen with drugs such as cyclophosphamide, actinomycin D and 5-fluorouracil (5-FU). There was a straight line log kill effect seen on both the normal and the malignant cells but with the cell killing effect being much greater in the malignant cell population.

At first inspection there did not appear to be any obvious correlation between the chemical structure and the mechanism of action of a drug and the type of dose response curve it produced. Two of the drugs in the class II grouping were antimetabolites, but one of the drugs, 5-FU, in the class III grouping was also an antimetabolite. A clue as to a possible basis for the different shaped survival curves was given by the fact that the tritiated thymidine used as one of the drugs yielded a class II-type dose response curve.

At the doses of the thymidine employed, the radioactive tritium in the compound was potent enough to kill any cell that commenced DNA

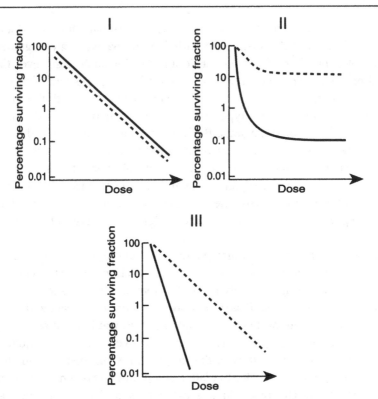

Fig. 2.10. The three classes of dose response curves seen for cancer chemotherapeutic agents. Each dose level of drug was given in divided doses every 6 hours for four doses. Surviving fractions for both normal and malignant cells were measured using spleen colony assays (see text for details): —, lymphoma stem cells; - - -, normal haematopoietic stem cells. (Adapted from Bruce, Meaker and Valeriote, 1966.)

synthesis and incorporated the thymidine into its DNA. Only cells in S phase would incorporate thymidine, which meant that those cells that commenced DNA synthesis during the '24 hour window' when the thymidine was being administered would undergo lethal injury. Likewise it was known that methotrexate acted primarily on cells entering S phase, as did ara-C. The drug vincristine was known to act primarily on the formation of the mitotic apparatus and would, therefore, exert its effects on cells passing through M. It appeared, therefore, that the plateau in the dose response curve in class II responses was caused by the presence of a subpopulation of cells that did not enter a vulnerable phase of the cell cycle during the duration of drug exposure. Further evidence supporting this hypothesis was obtained when the duration of exposure to the cytotoxic agents was increased to 48 hours. This produced a significantly greater fractional cell kill of both normal and malignant cells (Fig. 2.11).

Most of the class III agents were known to bind or damage DNA directly and were believed to exert their effects more or less uniformly throughout the cell cycle. The production of DNA lesions would then be proportional to the dose of drug, generating a log linear dose response curve. The inclusion of 5-FU in the class III category was initially puzzling as this drug was known to inhibit one of the key enzymes involved in DNA synthesis. However, at the high pulse doses employed in the experiments, 5-FU also inhibits RNA and protein synthesis, giving it a toxicity spectrum that would act throughout the entire cell cycle (Fig. 2.12).

The studies of Bruce and coworkers (1966) demonstrated for the first time that there was a significant differential toxic effect against malignant as opposed to normal cells. The basis for this differential effect was suggested by earlier studies of Till and McCulloch (1961), who had shown that in the normal 'steady state' condition of the bone marrow a high proportion of the colony-forming cells were not passing through the cell cycle but were in a special quiescent stage known as G_0, a so-called resting state which cells enter from G_1. If a toxic insult was given to the marrow (for example by radiation) then the G_0 cells would be stimulated to enter the cell cycle in order to replenish the diminished stem cell pool. As the newly recruited stems cells were now actively cycling, they would be vulnerable to further cytotoxic effect. When Bruce repeated his experiments on regenerating marrow he found the differential toxicity observed earlier had largely disappeared, with the normal cells now as sensitive as the lymphoma cells.

Bruce referred to the class II agents as *phase specific* because their site of action was primarily on one phase or stage of the cell cycle. The class III agents were designated as *cycle specific*, indicating their preferential toxicity for cells in the active stages of the cell cycle (but not G_0). Skipper subsequently modified this terminology, describing the class II agents as 'cell cycle stage specific' and the class III agents as 'cell cycle stage non-specific'. A term 'cycle active' has been used to describe those agents that primarily act on cells in cycle, but it really has no provenance with respect to the original experiments.

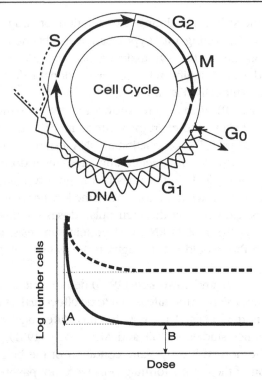

Fig. 2.11. Schematic representation for basis of class II (phase-specific) drug effect. The active form of ara-C interrupts DNA synthesis. The amount of DNA damage exceeds the repair capacity of the cell and apoptosis is initiated. During the duration of drug exposure (24 hours) the cohort of cells commencing DNA synthesis undergoes lethal damage. Cells that do not commence DNA synthesis during this time are not affected: - - -, normal haematopoietic stem cells; ——, lymphoma stem cells. A indicates the proportion of cells that sustain lethal damage and B the proportion of cells that do not enter S phase during the period of drug exposure (noncycling or slowing cycling cells).

Subsequently, van Putten in the Netherlands demonstrated that nitrogen mustard was actually a class III agent (van Putten, Lelieveld and Kram-Idsenga, 1972). The superimposition of the dose response curve for normal and malignant cells and the similarity to the effect of ionizing radiation was largely a coincidence relating to the relative resistance of the AKR lymphoma cells to nitrogen mustard. Thus the chemotherapeutic agents could be conveniently divided into two classes.

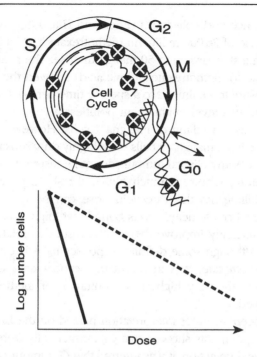

Fig. 2.12. Schematic representation for the class III (cycle-specific) drug effect. DNA molecules are damaged throughout the cell cycle. There is less damage with easier repair carried out in G_0 normal cells: - - -, normal cells; —, malignant cells. The number of DNA lesions produced will be proportional to dose. As the dose is increased more cells will sustain lethal injury (first-order kinetic log kill effect). The difference in log kill between normal and malignant cells reflects the fact that a greater amount of nonrepairable DNA damage is inflicted on the malignant cells than on the normal cells for a given dose of drug.

The Bruce experiments provided valuable insight into some of the processes involved in cancer chemotherapy, especially regarding the strategies that might be adopted to modify toxicity. Class II agents would provide a plateau in normal cell killing provided that the duration of exposure was kept to a short time interval. This suggested that it would be possible to escalate greatly the doses of those class II agents that did not have significant toxicity independent of their effect on dividing cells. Methotrexate being an analogue of a water-soluble vitamin (folic acid) was such a drug and it was found that it could be given in doses as much as 1000-fold greater than the standard doses employed.

For example, Price and colleagues (Price and Hill, 1983) were able to administer a dose of 20 000 milligram methotrexate in a 24 hour period compared with a standard 10 to 50 milligram dose. The availability of a specific antidote to methotrexate (folinic acid) allowed the duration of cytotoxic exposure to be limited to a specific time period. Escalating the dose of drug to this level might seem pointless as there would be no associated increase in killing of malignant cells. However, this would only be the case if the malignant cells were highly drug sensitive, like the AKR lymphoma. Many clinical tumours are quite resistant to methotrexate and, therefore, require a much higher threshold dose to start to produce cell killing. As this threshold dose can be reached without increasing normal cell toxicity, it was hoped that 'high-dose methotrexate' might significantly improve therapeutic results in relatively refractory tumours. Although some definite responses have been noted with high-dose methotrexate, it is apparent that cancer cells can become resistant to even the very highest concentration of methotrexate that can be employed.

There has been a further interpretation placed on the Bruce studies. Because the experiments showed that G_0 normal cells were very resistant to cytotoxic drug action, it was inferred that G_0 tumour cells likewise would be at least temporarily resistant to chemotherapy. However, it is noted that the Bruce experiments themselves provide little evidence for G_0 malignant stem cells. Virtually all of the lymphoma cells appeared to be in the active cell cycle mode. Whether or not this is a particular property of the AKR lymphoma and similar experimental tumours and not applicable to the behaviour of clinical malignancies is still uncertain.

Clinical tumours indeed contain many nondividing cells, but the great majority of these appear to be terminally differentiated cells or cells that have simply arrested in one part of the cell cycle but are not necessarily in G_0. Whether there are analogous states to the physiological G_0 condition that can be occupied by tumour cells is still not clearly established. One of the fundamental lesions that appears to be present in cancer is the relative inability of the cells to stop in G_1 and instead they continue on through the cell cycle. However, some tumour cells may have the capacity to enter some type of dormant or vegetative state, perhaps different from physiological G_0. Any tumour cells occupying this type of state would be 'kinetically resistant' and could present a barrier to drug-induced cure. However, this would be true primarily if treatment were confined to one or two applications of therapy; unless a period of dormancy were to persist for a very extended period of time, one would anticipate that as cells re-entered the division cycle they would again become vulnerable to chemotherapeutic effects. This is assuming that the cells were in other respects fundamentally sensitive to chemotherapy. The question of dormant states in tumours is an intriguing one. In tissue culture, cancer cells cease dividing when they have reached a concentration at which metabolites and growth factors become depleted. At this point, the cells begin dying at random points throughout the cell cycle. There is also some evidence that *in vivo* tumours that are 'dormant' may actually be in a state where proliferation is balanced by apoptosis so there is no net growth. If this has relevance to clinical malignancies then it has some important implications for the biology of the tumour when it resumes growth. We could expect that mutations and overall heterogeneity of the tumours would increase even if cell numbers were static (see also Chapter 6).

Summary and conclusions

The studies of Skipper, Schabel, Bruce and their colleagues provided clinicians with a much clearer model of the processes involved in cancer chemotherapy. Bruce's studies demonstrated that at least one type of resistance to anticancer drugs was related to the position in the division cycle that the cell occupied. This type of resistance appeared to be temporary in nature and contributed to the differential toxic effects of chemotherapy on normal versus malignant cells.

Skipper's work demonstrated that giving insufficient courses or doses of treatment could cause therapeutic failure, as would giving the treatments at too widely spaced intervals. Both these approaches resulted in the outgrowth of what was essentially a drug-sensitive neoplasm. This circumstance might be described as 'kinetic' escape, in which the net log kill was insufficient to control the malignancy. Solutions to these types of kinetic problem immediately suggested themselves. This required optimizing both the number and frequency of treatment courses without, at the same time, losing the therapeutic index provided by the differences in kinetic states between normal and malignant tissues.

Skipper also found evidence of a potentially more ominous problem. Cure of large tumour burdens was frequently prevented by the outgrowth of what appeared to be specific and permanently drug-resistant cells. The presence of these cells provided an additional rationale for the use of multiagent therapy, which, by this time, was being used at the clinical level. The logical question to be asked was 'what was the origin of these resistant cells and how could their impact be minimized?'.

In fact, the problem of drug-resistant cells in cancer had been recognized some years earlier and investigations had been done to determine the biological origin of these cells. As well, during the 1950s, the first studies of biochemical differences between drug-sensitive and drug-resistant cells were carried out.

However, it is to the question of the origin of resistant cells that we will next turn. A means of answering this question had been provided by Luria and Delbrück in 1943, in their studies of resistance in bacteria. This was followed in 1952 by the work of Law, who applied the Luria–Delbrück method to studying drug-resistant leukaemia cells in mice. Because of the importance of these studies, they will be explored in detail in Chapter 4.

References

Bruce, W.R. and van der Gaag, H. (1963). A quantitative assay for the number of murine lymphoma cells capable of proliferation *in vivo*. *Nature*, 199: 79–80.

Bruce, W.R., Meaker, B.E. and Valeriote, F.A. (1966). Comparison of normal hematopoietic and transplanted lymphoma colony forming cells to chemotherapeutic agents administered in vivo. *J. Nat. Cancer Inst.*, 37: 233–245.

Bush, R.S. and Hill, R.P. (1975). Biologic discussion of augmenting radiation effects and model systems. *Laryngoscope*, 85: 1119–1133. The first presentation that the authors are aware of in which a formal stem cell model of human cancer is presented.

Howard, A. and Pelc, S.R. (1953). Synthesis of deoxyribonucleic acid in normal and irradiated cells and its relation to chromosome breakage. *Heredity Suppl.*, 6: 261–273.

Hryniuk, W.M. and Bush, H. (1984). The importance of dose intensity in metastatic breast cancer. *J. Clin. Oncol.*, 2: 1281–1288.

Law, L.W. (1952). Origin of the resistance of leukemic cells to folic acid antagonists. *Nature*, 169: 628–629.

Luria, S.E. and Delbrück, M. (1943). Mutators of bacteria from virus sensitivity to virus resistance. *Genetics*, 28: 491–511.

MacKillop, W.J., Ciampi, A., Till, J.E. *et al.* (1983). A stem cell model of human tumour growth. Implication for tumour cell clonogenic assays. *J. Nat. Clin. Inst.*, 70: 9–16.

Price, L.A. and Hill, B.T. (1983). Safer cancer chemotherapy using a kinetically based experimental approach. *Mt Sinai J. Med.*, 52: 452–459.

Skipper, H.E., Schabel, F.M. Jr and Wilcox, W.S. (1964). Experimental evaluation of potential anti-cancer agents. XIII On the criteria and kinetics associated with 'Curability' of experimental leukemia. *Cancer Chemother.*, 35: 1–11. The classic paper by Skipper *et al.* that has provided a great deal of the basis of present day cytotoxic chemotherapy. The article is virtually of text book length and contains an enormous amount of supporting experimental data.

Till, J.E. and McCulloch, E.A. (1961). A direct measurement of the radiation sensitivity of normal mouse bone marrow cells. *Radiation Res.*, 14: 213–222.

Till, J.E., McCulloch, E.A. and Simonovitch, L. (1964). Stochastic model of stem cell proliferation based on growth of spleen colony forming cells. *Proc. Natl. Acad. Sci. USA*, 51: 29–36. The classic paper describing the process of renewal probability in haematopoietic stem cells.

van Putten, L.M., Lelieveld, P. and Kram-Idsenga, L.K.J. (1972). Cell cycle specificity and therapeutic effectiveness of cytostatic agents. *Cancer Chemother. Rep.*, 56: 691–700.

Further reading

Baserga, R., DeVita, V.T., Hellman, S.A. *et al.* (eds.) (1993). *Principles of Molecular Cell Biology of Cancer. Principles and Practice of Oncology*, pp. 60–66. Lippincott, Philadelphia, PA.

Buick, R.N. and MacKillop, W.J. (1981). Measurement of self renewal in culture of clonogenic cells from human ovarian carcinoma. *Br. J. Cancer*, 44: 349–355.

Counter, C.M., Hirte, H.W., Bacchetti, S. *et al.* (1994). Telomerase activity in human ovarian carcinoma. *Proc. Natl. Acad. Sci. USA*, 91: 2900–2904.

de Lange, T. (1994). Activation of telomerase in a human tumour. *Proc. Natl. Acad. Sci. USA*, 91: 2882–2885.

Hewitt, H.B. (1958). Studies of the dissemination and quantitative transplantation of a lymphocytic leukemia of CBA mice. *Br. J. Cancer*, 12: 378–401.

Lindenboim, L., Diamond, R., Rothenberg, E. and Stein, R. (1995). Apoptosis induced by serum deprivation of PC12 cells is not preceded by growth arrest and can occur at each phase of the cell cycle. *Cancer Res.*, 55: 1242–1247.

Norton, L. and Simon, R. (1977). Tumour size, sensitivity to therapy and design of treatment schedules. *Cancer Treat.*, 61: 1307–1317.

O'Reilly, M.S., Holmgren, L., Chen, C. *et al.* (1996). Angiostatin induces and sustains dormancy of human primary tumors in mice. *Nature Med.*, 2: 689–692.

Schackney, S.E., McCormack, G.W. and Cuchural, G.J. Jr (1978). Growth rate patterns of solid tumours and their relation to responsiveness to therapy; an analytic review. *Ann. Intern. Med.*, 89: 107–121.

Steel, G.G. and Lamerton, L.F. (1968). Cell population kinetics and chemotherapy in human tumour cell kinetics. *Natl. Cancer Inst. Mono.*, 30: 29–50.

Swan, G.W. (1977). *Some Current Mathematical Topics in Cancer Research*, pp. 1–6, 71–83. University Microfilms International, Ann Arbor, MI. A detailed monograph on several aspects relating to the growth and proliferative properties of cancer cell populations. This is a highly specialized text for readers with a substantial mathematical background.

Wheldon, T.E. (1988). Models of tumour growth. In *Mathematical Models in Cancer Research*, pp. 63–89. Hilger, Bristol. A very useful account of a number of models of tumour growth and radiation and chemotherapy effect. Although there is a considerable amount of mathematics in the text, the author avoids using higher mathematical theory and the development of the mathematical models is well explained by the accompanying text. This is probably the most accessible of the mathematical model texts in the oncology area.

Whitmore, G.F. and Till, J.E. (1964). Quantitation of cellular radiobiological responses. *Annu. Rev. Nucl. Sci.*, 14: 347–375.

3

Molecular aspects of drug resistance

3.1 Introduction

There are approximately 60 different chemical compounds generally available for the treatment of cancer (not including hormones or biological response modifiers). They are of diverse structure and from a variety of sources. They do not readily fit into a single classification system and are usually described partly on the basis of their chemical structure, partly on their primary source (fungi, plant, etc.) and partly on what is thought to be their general mechanism of action (antimetabolite, alkylating agent, etc.) (Table 3.1). We can generalize by stating that all of the drugs appear to exert their therapeutic effect by interfering with the processes involved in cell division. This interference results in the cell being physically disrupted or rendered permanently sterile. We can further say that cancer cells have the potential to become resistant to any of the drugs in our inventory and the cell can, moreover, express resistance to a great many agents simultaneously. Although we are not aware of the experiment actually having been done, it seems more than probable that an individual cancer cell could display resistance to all 60 available drugs concurrently. As we will see, this capacity to express resistance to many agents is, in part, related to the fact that there are a large number of mechanisms that once expressed by the cell will generate broad degrees of cellular resistance.

It would be well beyond the scope of this book to discuss in any detail the molecular changes that have been described for all of the various cytotoxic agents. However, we will mention the general processes involved in drug action and how these may be modified in the drug-resistant state.

Table 3.1 *The main groupings of common anticancer drugs with some representative agents in each class*[a]

Classes	Examples
Alkylating agents	Mustard derivatives: nitrogen mustard, cyclophosphamide, melphelan, iphosphamide, etc. Nitrosourea derivatives: bischloroethylnitrosourea (BCNC), ciscyclohexylnitrosourea (CCNU) Platinum compounds: cisplatinum, carboplatin Imidazole carboxamide compounds (DTIC) Miscellaneous compounds: Thio tepa Procarbazine Trietixylene melamine
Antimetabolites	Folic acid antagonists: aminopterin, methotrexate, trimetrexate Purine antagonists: 6-mercaptopurine, 6-thioguanine, chlorodeoxyadenosine Pyrimidine antagonists: 5-fluorouracil (5-FU), 5-fluorodeoxyuridine (5-FUDR), cytosine arabinoside (ara-C), gemcytabine, fludarabine
Natural products	Antibiotics: doxorubicin, daunorubicin, mitomycin C, actinomycin D, bleomycin Plant alkaloids: vincristine, vinblastine, paclitaxel (taxol), camptothecin
Synthetic agents	Hydroxyurea, lonidamine, mitoxantrone
Hormonal agents	Androgens, oestrogens, antioestrogens (tamoxifen), antiandrogens (cyproterone)
Vitamin analogues	Vitamin A anlogues (retinoids), vitamin D analogues

[a] Many of the compounds could fit in more than one category (e.g. mitomycin C is an antibiotic that functions as an alkylating agent). The full list of anticancer drugs that have had at least preliminary testing in patients could be considerably larger than this.

3.2 Genetic alterations associated with drug resistance

It is readily apparent how a mutation that results in a loss of function in a protein could mediate drug resistance. The mutated protein may be smaller than the normal one because the mutant gene results in termination of RNA transcription before the complete code for the protein is read out. The truncated protein may have greatly diminished function or may be nonfunctional. As there are two alleles for each gene, loss of 50% function may not be a lethal mutation for the cell but may be sufficient to reduce significantly the rate of transport of a drug (if the protein involved is a receptor) or reduce the rate of metabolic conversion of a drug to its active form. A point mutation occurring at the binding site of a transport protein or an enzyme involved in drug metabolism may greatly diminish the affinity between the drug and the protein. The loss of affinity may be much less for the normal substrate so that the mutant cell is at only a small disadvantage with respect to normal metabolism and has acquired a huge selective advantage in any environment where the particular toxic drug is present.

If mutations affect both alleles causing loss of function, the viability of the cell will depend on whether or not this constitutes a lethal impairment. Because many tumour cells have chromosomal abnormalities (rearrangements, translocations, deletions or actual loss of entire chromosome) the cell may be hemizygous (one copy) for a particular allele. A single mutation would then suffice to delete completely the function of certain genes. The enzymes that are involved in converting many antimetabolites to their active nucleotide form are part of the so-called nucleic acid salvage pathway, which allows cells to scavenge nucleic acid precursors from both the internal and external environment efficiently. These enzymes are not essential for viability, however, as nucleic acids can be built up from much simpler molecules. A cell with a deficient scavenging system would be at a slight disadvantage compared with the wild type and, therefore, could be expected to occur only infrequently in the unselected population. Exposure to drugs such as ara-C or 5-FU would provide a powerful selection pressure on the cells and now the 'disadvantaged' salvage-deficient cells would be favoured as they would not convert the drugs into their lethal active form.

Many types of drug resistance are associated with an actual gain of function of a particular protein. This will be apparent with the various systems that are involved with detoxification of a drug, with proteins that are involved in moving the drug out of the cell or with proteins involved in actually repairing the damage that the drug inflicts on the cell macromolecules. Although these gain-of-function mutations may involve the structural gene itself, producing a mutant protein with enhanced functional capacity, it more often involves mutations that regulate transcription of the structural gene. A common genetic lesion involves a structural

gene being translocated by a chromosomal mutation that moves
the gene to an abnormal site. Here it may be adjacent to a different
promoter gene than normally functions to regulate the structural gene.
Under these circumstances, the gene may be continuously stimulated to
function.

Increased function of a gene can also be mediated through an
increase in gene copy number to greater than the normal complement
of two. This arises through abnormal duplication of the gene sequence
such that several copies of the gene may now be present in an expanded
region of the chromosome. This process of gene amplification is commonly associated with certain types of drug resistance; the genetic
instability that underlies it appears to be essentially unique to the malignant state. Amplified genes are virtually never observed in normal cells.

The neoplastic cell population will be continuously generating a large
range of genotypes. This will include both gain-of-function and loss-of-
function mutations. A large number of the cell's genes will be affected,
and not simply those associated with drug resistance. Many genotypes
will yield phenotypes that are little different from the wild type and,
therefore, will be co-selected along with the wild type, producing a
group of genotypes around the common or consensus type. Eigen
(1992) refers to this population of closely related genotypes as a
'quasi-species'. It is the quasi-species that is acted upon by the environment. As it may consist of many closely related individuals, the 'pool' of
phenotypes that the environment acts upon is large. This will ensure that
the rate of evolution of new better adapted forms will be quite rapid. A
neutral mutation may persist as part of the quasi-species until exposed to
a cytotoxic agent that now selects for it and renders it the dominant
phenotype. The evolutionary process will continue with a new quasi-
species 'condensing' around the new wild phenotype. In time, a better
adapted mutant will displace the first and so on. Phenomenologically
this will present itself as a very rapid emergence and selection for drug-
resistant forms under the impact of chemotherapeutic exposure.

The simple diagrams usually used to illustrate the mutational process,
in which there is one distinctly marked mutant cell against a background
of homogeneous normal cells represents a considerable oversimplification of the actual circumstance that occurs in real systems. The genetic
processes generate an enormous amount of diversity, with many genotypes probably making up what constitutes a single phenotype. The
process is dynamic and continuously changing; when a strong selection

pressure is applied, there are many closely related variant forms that undergo selection. In reviewing the molecular changes that are associated with various drug-resistant states, it is convenient to discuss these changes as though they occurred in isolation from a great many other concurrent changes that must be happening within the cell. However, a single class of phenotype, which might be defined operationally as the ability to survive a 24 hour exposure to doxorubicin at a concentration of 10^{-6} M, would almost certainly be made up of a number of separate genotypes with differing mechanisms of resistance but all having the common property of being able to survive selection by the drug under defined conditions of stringency.

3.3   Cancer chemotherapy: methods of administration

Anticancer agents are most commonly administered by the intravenous or oral route. For special circumstances, some agents may be given by direct injection into a body cavity (intrapleural, intra-abdominal, intra-vesicle or into the cerebrospinal fluid). Much less commonly, agents can be given intra-arterially or even intralymphatically. Some agents can be applied topically and some can be given intramuscularly or by direct injection into the tumour mass.

Once the drug enters the systemic circulation, it becomes distributed throughout the entire body (less efficiently into tissues such as the central nervous system, eyes and the testes). Some drugs may require metabolic conversion in the liver, but most agents are taken up by the cells in the same molecular form as they were administered. There is no preferential localization of drug in the area of the tumour although methods to alter this are being investigated (i.e. antibody labelling, liposomal encapsulation). Given the complexity of the pharmacology of these agents, it is remarkable that it has been possible to extrapolate from *in vitro* experiments to the degree that this has been done. This would reinforce the assumption that it is the drug–cancer cell interaction that predominates in clinical chemotherapy.

3.4   Drug uptake

Anticancer drugs gain access to the interior of the cell by either an active or a passive transport process. In passive transport, drug molecules diffuse across the cell membrane and this generally requires a high extracellular drug concentration and the absence of a strong electrical charge on the drug molecule. Compounds that are fairly soluble in lipid can more easily move across the cell membrane, which has a high lipid content.

Compounds that are ionized and relatively soluble in water have a more difficult time crossing the cell membrane (less at extremely high concentrations), as they have to move across a thermodynamic barrier that exists in the form of the hydrophobic hydrocarbon region of cell membranes, the first of which encountered is the plasma membrane. Movement of such molecules is facilitated by the drug binding to a special transport molecule on the cell surface, which then translocates the drug molecule to the cell's interior. This translocation may require an expenditure of energy by the cell. There is a large variety of such transport proteins (or receptors) on the cell surface that have evolved for the purposes of transporting essential nutrients and growth factors into the cell. The cytotoxic drug may be sufficiently similar to a normal substrate that it can latch onto the receptor and be transported into the cell. These active transport systems are designed to move molecules against both concentration and electrical gradients and will transport substrates even when the substance is present in a very low extracellular concentration. Even if the drug has relatively low affinity for the receptor it will generally be present in much greater concentration than the substrate and thus effectively utilize the transport system.

Resistance to a drug may be associated with mutant forms of the receptor such that affinity for the normal substrate is retained but there is a greatly reduced affinity for the drug. There may be reductions in the number of receptor molecules on the cell surface, which will also impede the rate of influx of drug. Both types of change in receptors can occur concurrently, having the effect of significantly reducing the net intracellular concentration of drug. This will, in turn, reduce the probability of interaction between the drug and its intracellular targets.

3.5 Drug efflux

In addition to the above processes for mediating drug entry into the cell, there are some extremely important mechanisms for drug efflux out of the cell interior. The net intracellular drug concentration will, accordingly, be reduced. These mechanisms are present in many normal cells but may have increased expression in a number of types of tumour cell.

They clearly will have a protective effect against drug-induced injury and they are responsible for mediating resistance to a wide variety of antineoplastic agents. The condition where a cell expresses resistance to a variety of types of anticancer drug through a single discrete mechanism is known as *multidrug resistance* (MDR) (see p. 68).

3.6   Drug–target interaction

Once a drug has achieved a critical threshold level of intracellular concentration, it will interact with a great range of cellular macromolecules. These include enzymes that are involved in the synthesis of nucleic acid precursors, proteins involved in the structure of the mitotic apparatus, enzymes involved in the synthesis and structural integrity of DNA, enzymes involved in repairing damaged DNA and, finally, direct binding to DNA itself, impairing its function. There are other targets as well, including enzymes involved in energy transfer and proteins that participate in the very complex signal pathways for both stimulating and suppressing cell division. Many of the experimental data in the literature deal with the great variety of potential drug targets and the changes in these targets that can generate drug resistance. We can say generally that a cell may become resistant to a particular drug if the amount of the target molecule is altered (both increases and decreases may mediate resistance) or if a change in the protein structure itself results in reduced affinity between drug and target.

3.7   Intracellular drug activation

Some drugs require further biochemical modification before they are able to function. Typically, one sees this with the group of antimetabolite drugs that are analogues of DNA precursors (e.g. 5-FU, ara-C, etc.). These molecules are virtually inert until they undergo a series of steps to convert them into the nucleotide form (e.g. 5-FU to 5-fluorodeoxyuridine monophosphate (5-FdUMP)). Their close chemical similarity to the normal nucleotide allows them to inhibit one or other of the enzymes involved in DNA synthesis. In the case of 5-FdUMP, this involves inhibition of the enzyme thymidylate synthase (TS), which catalyzes the final step in the synthesis of thymidine from precursor molecules. Resistance to 5-FU could arise from mutations altering the affinity site in the TS molecule or increased expression of TS, which would, in turn, require a greater intracellular concentration of drug to achieve inhibition. Resistance to 5-FU will also occur if there is loss of cellular capacity to synthesize the active form of the drug. If there is complete loss of function in this synthetic pathway then the loss of sensitivity to 5-FU will be virtually complete. Similar gain- or loss-of-function mutations will affect the other pyrimidine and purine analogue antimetabolites (e.g. ara-C, 6-mercaptopurine, fludarabine, etc.).

Mutations affecting the function of these types of compound are common, but unlike the MDR phenotypes, the resistance profile produced tends to be confined to the specific drug or at least to the defined class to which it belongs. This potentially makes the concurrent use of antimetabolites with alkylating agents or natural product compounds attractive combination protocols.

3.8 Intracellular detoxification

There are a number of enzyme systems within the cell that have the capacity to detoxify drugs that contain very reactive chemical groups (such as alkylating agents) or to break down the active oxidizing compounds (such as hydrogen peroxide) which are produced by the action of a variety of cytotoxic agents. One of the most important of theses detoxification processes is the glutathione (GSH) system, which includes at least two enzymes: GSH S-transferase and GSH peroxidase. GSH S-transferase binds GSH to the reactive alkylating groups in drugs such as nitrogen mustard and cyclophosphamide preventing them from reacting with or cross-linking DNA. Increased activity of the GSH system is felt to constitute another mechanism of MDR. Along with the drug-effluxing proteins, the GSH system appears to have evolved as a cellular protection mechanism against a wide variety of cell poisons.

3.9 DNA-binding drugs

A substantial number of antineoplastic agents produce their cytotoxic effects by directly binding to DNA or by interacting with enzymes that are involved with maintaining the structural integrity of DNA. The drugs involved include all of the alkylating-type agents (mustard derivatives, nitrosoureas, platinum compounds, etc.) plus a number of natural product substances such as actinomycin D and bleomycin. Collectively, these compounds constitute by far the most widely used clinical agents at the present time.

A great deal is known about these drugs in terms of their specific mechanisms of action as well as many of the molecular changes that are associated with drug resistance. In the case of drugs that directly bind chemically to DNA there exists a complex biochemical machinery for recognizing that DNA has been damaged and then repairing the lesion. The repair process consists of identifying the region that has been damaged, excising the abnormal segment then replacing the segment with newly synthesized DNA elements. These excision–repair systems are remarkable for their sensitivity and accuracy. The fidelity of the repair process has been estimated to be accurate to 1 part in 10^{10}. One class of alkylating agents, the nitrosoureas, link to a specific atom (O^6) in the guanine base of DNA. A specific enzyme system, O^6-guanylmethyl transferase efficiently removes the nitrosourea adduct from the DNA, thus preventing cytotoxicity. Cells that have a significant methyl transferase activity are known as the Mer$^+$ phenotype and those lacking it as Mer$^-$. Unfortunately it appears that most human cancer cells are Mer$^+$, whereas many mouse tumours appear to be Mer$^-$. This could partly explain the fact that the nitrosourea compounds that were dramatically effective in treating mouse tumours in the preclinical screening tests have been moderately disappointing in human chemotherapy, with their use confined to only a few tumour types.

Tumour cells that display reduced sensitivity to alkylating agent damage have frequently been found to have an enhanced capacity for carrying out DNA repair. Although the capacity of the tumour cells to repair damage is substantial, the accuracy of the repair may be diminished. Thus the chemotherapeutic agents may aggravate the process of mutations occurring in nonlethally damaged cells.

3.10   The topoisomerase system

Two enzyme systems that are vitally involved with maintaining the three-dimensional structure of DNA during RNA synthesis and DNA replication are topoisomerase I and topoisomerase II. Topoisomerase I produces single-strand breaks in DNA to allow the DNA molecule to unwind itself and then the ends of the cut strands are ligated. Topoisomerase II carries out single- and double-strand breaks, which permit more complex uncoiling of the loops of DNA. This permits RNA to be synthesized on the coding strand of DNA as well as allowing orderly separation of the DNA strands during replication. A variety of drugs bind to the topoisomerase–DNA complex, stabilizing it and preventing the broken strands from being joined. Inhibitors of topoisomerase II include doxorubicin, etoposide and teniposide. Inhibitors of topoisomerase I include analogues of the plant alkaloid camptothecin. Resistance to agents of this category have been associated with mutant forms of the enzyme that are still able to carry out their biochemical functions but have reduced affinity for the cytotoxic drug.

3.11   The multidrug-resistant phenotype

In the early 1970s investigators noted that cell lines that had been selected for resistance to one class of natural product anticancer agents (e.g. vincristine) would also display resistance to a number of other drugs (e.g. doxorubicin, actinomycin D, etoposide) even though the cell had never been previously exposed to these agents. This phenomenon was called 'pleiotropic' resistance and it was found to be commonly present in cells that had been selected by exposure to a large number of certain types of antineoplastic agents.

The resistance was not universal, however, and the cell lines retained sensitivity to alkylating agents, antimetabolites and a few types of natural product compound (e.g. bleomycin). The drugs that were associated with pleiotropic resistance did tend to have a few features in common. They had large molecular weights and had complex organic ring structures. They were either directly derived from some natural product (fungi, plants) or semisynthetic analogues of a natural product compound. Aside from that they had little in common They were chemically very dissimilar and had different loci of action inside the cell.

The term pleiotropic resistance has started to be dropped in favour of the term multidrug resistance (MDR). The MDR phenotype refers to any cell that can express resistance simultaneously to many different agents as a consequence of a single biochemical change. *Multilevel resistance* (MLR) should be reserved for cells that express a number of different drug resistance mechanisms concurrently. This latter phenomenon implies a sequence of discrete mutations rather than one mutation producing a broad degree of resistance.

MDR associated with P-gp

In 1976 Juliano and Ling identified a cell surface protein, of 170 000 molecular weight, that was associated with the pleiotropic resistance phenomenon. Designated P-glycoprotein (P-gp), this molecule was shown to function as a transporter for a variety of molecular structures from the interior of the cell. P-gp turns out to be a member of a family of structurally related proteins that has been strongly conserved across many species. Known collectively as ABC proteins (ABC: ATP-binding cassette), these molecules have an affinity site that will accept a wide variety of large-molecular-weight compounds. ATP also binds to the protein and provides energy that permits the translocation of the bound molecule to the outside of the cell. P-gp is coded for by a gene designated *mdr-1*. P-gp is found to be expressed at low levels in a number of normal cell types (colon, adrenal cortex, renal tubule) but much higher levels of expression are seen in a variety of tumours, especially those which have regrown after previous treatment by drugs that are known to be substrates for P-gp. Direct measurement of drug efflux in P-gp-positive cells can readily demonstrate the capacity of the P-gp to lower significantly the intracellular concentration of the cytotoxic drug. Transfection of *mdr-1* to P-gp-negative drug-sensitive cells will convert the cell into a P-gp-positive drug-resistant one. The cells will display a pattern of resistance typical of the MDR state.

Preliminary analysis in tumours such as neuroblastoma and large cell lymphoma indicate that patients whose tumour cells stain strongly positive for P-gp have a significantly worse outcome than those who are negative at the outset of treatment. In lymphoma, P-gp positivity presumably predicts for an increased probability of other drug-resistance mechanisms but does not completely preclude a favourable response to chemotherapy as some of these P-gp-positive patients are cured. Since lymphoma protocols contain some drugs that are not affected by P-gp, the presumption is that this may be sufficient to cure a few patients.

Interestingly, while P-gp-positive cells in experimental systems display resistance to the broad range of P-gp substrates, the highest order of resistance is seen with the drug that was used to select for the resistance in the first place. That is, if doxorubicin was used as a selecting agent then the cells will display greater resistance towards doxorubicin than vincristine or etoposide. If vincristine is the selecting agent then the cells will display more resistance to it and so on. This is probably explained by the fact that the drug-resistant cells have a complex phenotype, with increased P-gp being only one of the mechanisms present.

The MDR state associated with P-gp is often referred to as 'classical' MDR in recognition that it was the first type of broad-range resistance characterized. There have been a number of other mechanisms discovered that can also generate MDR and these are known collectively as 'nonclassical' or 'atypical' MDR.

MRP-associated MDR

Recently an ABC protein belonging to the same family as P-gp has been discovered in human cancer cells that display MDR but which are negative for P-gp. This new protein has been designated MRP (multiresistance protein), has a molecular weight of 190 000 and appears to function similarly to P-gp. However, cells can express MRP without expressing P-gp and vice versa. Likewise, cells may express both proteins concurrently. MRP-positive cells display resistance to many of the same compounds as P-gp-positive cells. However, this MDR phenotype appears to correlate more with altered intracellular drug distribution rather than the reduced drug uptake in resistant tumours that is observed for tumour cells overexpressing P-gp. Nonetheless, the underlying mechanism of MRP-related drug resistance is comparable to that arising from P-gp in as much as it reduces the level of drug at the site of antitumour action.

Glutathione-associated MDR

The glutathione transferase and glutathione peroxidase systems have been associated with resistance to many of the alkylating agent class of drug as well as to certain natural product compounds such as doxorubicin and bleomycin. In some instances, it has been shown to be possible to restore sensitivity to these drugs by prior treatment of the cells with some drugs, such as buthionine sulphoxamine, which deplete the cells of their intracellular glutathione content. Some investigators have suggested that the glutathione system may be coordinately expressed with P-gp as part of a general protective cell system against foreign toxins. Interestingly, MRP appears to function in normal cells as a transporter of glutathione conjugates, suggesting a more general correlation between detoxifying and transport-based resistance mechanisms.

Topoisomerase II-associated MDR

Mutations resulting in reduced activity of topoisomerase II or alterations in the drug-binding site in the enzyme have been described.
These changes can produce resistance to the drugs that bind to the
topoisomerase II–DNA complex, (doxorubicin, etoposide, teniposide).
The binding of the drug to the enzyme basically stabilizes the enzyme–
DNA complex so that the DNA, which has then been cleaved by the
enzyme, can now no longer be joined together. As with other types of
MDR, changes in the topoisomerase-II system may occur independently or concurrently with other types of MDR. Most of the compounds that are topoisomerase-II inhibitors are also affected by P-gp
expression. Research is actively being pursued to establish which
mechanisms may predominate in which particular type of tumour.
Breast cancer, for example, only infrequently seems to express P-gp
strongly but more often displays alterations in topoisomerase-II.

DNA repair-associated MDR

The complex system of DNA excision and repair enzymes may display
enhanced activity, which will significantly increase resistance to many of
the alkylating agent type of drug. Enhanced capacity to repair various
types of DNA lesion may allow the cell to remain viable even though
considerable DNA damage has been inflicted through drug action.

3.12   The relationship between apoptosis and drug resistance

The discovery of so many categories of MDR has been a somewhat
disconcerting finding. A single mutational event could result in resistance to a significant number of potent therapeutic agents at one step.
It does help explain, however, how tumour cells are able to display
resistance to so many drugs so rapidly. The occurrence of 5 or 10
mutations in the right place could neutralize most of our useful agents.
It means that as far as the tumour cell is concerned we are dealing with
many fewer discrete drugs than the simple number in our inventory
would suggest. However, it does also suggest that if one or two of the
resistance mechanisms can be modulated, or disabled, sensitivity to a
large number of drugs will be restored.

If the problems of MDR were not enough, recent studies point to another whole level at which broad categories of drug resistance may occur. This new evidence is of great significance because it not only explains a number of questions about the fundamental nature of drug resistance and its relationship to neoplastic state but it also provides a unifying theory as to how anticancer agents actually kill the tumour cell.

The work that has been carried out on programmed cell death (apoptosis) has provided a link between chemotherapy effect and the cancerous state. The gene for p53 plays a key role in regulating the movement of cells through the division cycle. At a point in G_1 p53 initiates a check program that, in effect, assesses the integrity of the cellular DNA. If any damage is detected then repair processes are commenced and further movement through the cell cycle is stopped until the repair is completed. If, however, the amount of genetic damage is above a threshold value where it cannot be repaired effectively, then the p53 protein signals the apoptosis sequence to begin (Fig. 3.1).

A series of chemical and morphological changes then begins that is characteristic of the apoptosis process. The chromatin in the cell nucleus becomes condensed and 'clumps' in a characteristic manner. Blebs form in the cell cytoplasm and begin fragmenting off. Molecular studies carried out at this time reveal that the DNA has become split up into fragments of a characteristic size, which are then encapsulated by cell nuclear material. The final destructive events in the cell are associated with an influx of calcium ions and the generation of highly reactive oxygen species. Internal cell membranes are disrupted and cell dissolution proceeds. The cytoplasmic and nuclear fragments are then phagocytosed by tissue macrophages. The whole sequence typically occurs rapidly (in less than an hour) and is not associated with any inflammatory response in the surrounding tissues. This helps to distinguish apoptosis from other types of cell injury and death reaction such as necrosis, which typically causes surrounding inflammation as well as usually affecting a large number of contiguous cells.

There appear to be a number of routes whereby apoptosis can be accessed and some of these occur independently of p53 function. However, the importance of p53-dependent apoptosis appears to lie with the fact that the p53 pathway is initiated at relatively low levels of DNA damage.

A cellular oncogene designated bcl-2 (so named because it was initially found in a B cell lymphoma) appears to function not by providing

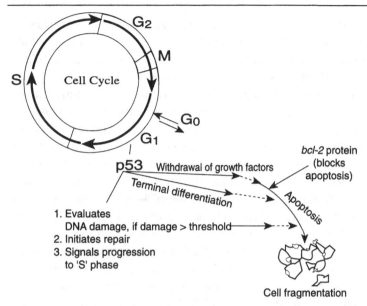

Fig. 3.1. The events of the cell cycle are shown in association with the function of p53 in evaluating DNA integrity and in signalling apoptosis. This is a greatly simplified diagram as there are many other factors and gene products that regulate passage through the cell cycle or initiate apoptosis. Interference with the *bcl-2* product favours stem cell self-renewal over differentiation. In normal cells *bcl-2* function is finely regulated; however, in a variety of malignancies *bcl-2* is continuously and inappropriately expressed.

positive growth signals but by inhibiting apoptosis. *bcl-2* is part of a complex system that coordinately acts to regulate apoptosis. The *bax* family of genes functions to oppose *bcl-2*, and it appears to be the *bcl-2/bax* ratio that is important in determining whether or not a cell undergoes apoptosis. Although *bcl-2* overexpression is a common alteration associated with malignancy, it should not be assumed that somehow *bcl-2* is a 'bad thing'. It is the inappropriate expresson of *bcl-2* that causes problems. The normally functioning protein product is essential for normal growth and development. So-called *bcl-2* knock-out mice, homozygous *bcl-2* (−/−) although viable at birth are prone to a number of serious congenital defects and early death owing to excessive apoptosis in a number of tissues and organs. It has been suggested that the *bcl-2* protein product functions as an antioxidant preventing the damage associated with oxygen species release. There appears to be homologues of the *bcl-2* protein in certain species of primitive bacteria, suggesting to some authors that the *bcl-2* family evolved very early in the history of life as a protectant against the developing oxygen atmosphere on the earth. (Interestingly, p53 does not appear to have a homologue in bacteria and protozoa, suggesting that it may have evolved much later when complex multicellular organisms appeared.) In normal cells, *bcl-2* is part of a complex pathway that coordinately opposes or promotes the apoptosis sequence. When apoptosis is suppressed, cells are in effect moved continuously through the cell cycle. This drives cell proliferation and self-renewal. When *bcl-2* is downregulated, differentiation and/or apoptosis is favoured. We can see, therefore that the p53–*bcl-2* system is part of the process of self-renewal and cell differentiation. It becomes easier to see how dysfunction of this system can contribute to the development of malignancy. Further, there appear to be complex interactions among the various oncogenes, tumour suppressor genes and other genes that mediate drug resistance. It has been found, for instance, that mutant p53 can interact with the promoter gene for MDR-1, producing increased expression of the gene and increased intracellular P-gp.

Members of the *ras* oncogene family, which do provide positive growth signals, also may produce increased resistance to certain antineoplastic agents. Transfection of *ras* into cisplatin-sensitive cells confers cisplatin resistance, although the precise mechanism is uncertain at this time.

In addition to the role played by tumour suppressor genes such as p53 and oncogenes that block apoptosis such as *bcl-2*, a number of the oncogenes provide positive growth signals and also influence drug sensitivity. The c-*myc* oncogene, which provides growth signals to the cell, will at the same time sensitize cells to apoptosis induction if certain essential growth factors are reduced. c-*myc* is constitutively overexpressed in certain lymphomas owing to a chromosomal mutation that sees the gene being translocated to a different chromosome where it comes under the influence of a promoter gene. On its own this change might produce an overproliferating clone of lymphoid cells that would be very sensitive to chemotherapy. However, the fully developed lymphoma tends also to be associated with *bcl-2* overexpression, which prevents apoptosis and at the same time favours stem cell proliferation.

Because chemotherapeutic agents often produce direct genotoxic damage they are potent initiators of p53-dependent apoptosis. Other types of cellular damage (e.g. damage to the mitotic spindle) can also initiate apoptosis, and these may, or may not, be mediated by the p53 gene. The G_2/M boundary in the cell cycle appears to be another critical point where DNA or chromosomal damage is repaired or an apoptosis-like sequence is commenced (sometimes referred to as 'mitotic cata-strophe'). Certain drugs and radiation may produce this effect, which appears to be independent of p53-associated apoptosis. A general sequence of chemotherapy effect may be: (a) transport into the cell, (b) direct or indirect damage to DNA or the mitotic apparatus, (c) apoptosis triggered if the drug-induced damage cannot be repaired. Since it appears that chemotherapeutic drugs generate cell killing by inducing apoptosis, this may constitute the final common pathway for many anti-cancer agents.

Supporting evidence for believing that p53-dependent apoptosis is an important determinant of drug sensitivity has been obtained by studying tumour cell lines that express different levels of p53 (Lowe *et al.*, 1993). Cells that had two functional alleles for p53 (i.e. p53 +/+) displayed marked sensitivity to a variety of antineoplastic agents plus radiation, whereas the p53−/−cells were both drug and radiation resistant. Cells heterozygous for p53 displayed an intermediate level of resistance between the two types. Transfection of normal p53 into p53 null cells restored drug and radiation sensitivity.

Other studies have suggested that p53 status on its own could influence drug resistance without there being any other (apparent) molecular changes producing drug resistance. It is shown that cells would express resistance to 5-FU if they were p53 negative even if the rest of the 5-FU pathway was intact (as measured by inhibition of thymidylate synthesis).

The gene for p53 is only one part of a complex signalling pathway that controls movement through the cell cycle and provides signals for apoptosis. Presumably alteration in any of the genes that participate in this pathway could influence drug sensitivity. There are, as well, the p53-independent pathways that can also signal apoptosis and could potentially influence drug sensitivity.

Given the frequency with which p53 is mutated in human cancer, it is not surprising that many malignancies are characterized by relative resistance to chemotherapy. However, it would be a mistake to assume that because these mutations are widespread most human malignancies are fundamentally untreatable by cytotoxic agents. Most types of cancer are at least moderately sensitive to chemotherapy even if they cannot be cured. Even sensitive (and curable) tumours could be expected to have at least small subpopulations of p53-negative cells. The p53 status can be viewed as *one* of the important functions influencing drug resistance but, on its own, it will not generate the levels of resistance seen in highly selected human cells. This issue will be revisited when we come to consider the question of intrinsic resistance in Chapters 6 and 9.

It is interesting to note that we can see a relationship between apoptosis and the birth/death mathematical processes that will be described later. The molecular equivalents to the birth/death process can be seen in the positive growth signals provided by cellular oncogenes (birth) and the differentiation or death signals provided by the tumour suppressor genes such as p53. Just as the mathematical equations suggest that cancer must arise from an imbalance between cell birth and cell death, laboratory studies indicate that tumours develop through mutations that negatively affect the function of the cell death/differentiation genes or through inappropriate overexpression of the cell birth genes (oncogenes). Many cancers appear to have mutations in both components of the growth system, leading to a general genetic instability and ultimately all of the phenomena that we associate with cancer: excessive growth, loss of normal differentiated function and the acquisition of such properties as invasiveness and capacity to metastasize.

3.13   Drug-resistance modulation

The discovery of P-gp-mediated MDR provided impetus to attempt to develop drugs that would specifically disable the resistance mechanism, thereby restoring at one step sensitivity to many different therapeutic agents. Tsuro in Japan (1983) found that calcium channel-blocking agents such as verapamil could interfere with the binding of the antitumour agent to the drug affinity site on the P-gp molecule. It was possible to demonstrate in *in vitro* systems that this would significantly impair drug efflux, resulting in the maintenance of a cytotoxic intracellular concentration of the drug. These finding have stimulated an extensive search for drugs that would be more effective than verapamil and less toxic. A number of different classes of compound have been found including such diverse agents as chlorpromazine, tamoxifen, medroxyprogesterone and quinidine. The most potent agents discovered so far are analogues of the naturally occurring immunosuppressive agent cyclosporine. Some moderate degrees of restoration of drug sensitivity have been seen in preliminary clinical trials, but so far dramatic responses have not been observed. This may not be surprising given the probable multifactorial basis for drug resistance, in advanced tumours at least. For example, there are at least two independent mechanisms for resistance to doxorubicin (probably more). Even if P-gp-positive cells are effectively modulated, alterations in topoisomerase II could still generate drug resistance and the effect of the modulator would be significantly diminished. An unanswered question at this time is whether the *earlier* use of the modulator together with P-gp class cytotoxic agents would retard the development of resistance. In any case, it is probable that successful drug-resistance modulation will require the simultaneous use of at least two or three agents to deal with the common forms of MDR. There will be a need for more potent and less toxic modulators, especially if they are to be used in combination. Interestingly, antineoplastic agents such as doxorubicin, etoposide, vincristine, etc., which are good P-gp substrates, do not appear to modulate resistance to one another. This suggests that the antineoplastic drug-binding site on the P-gp molecule is not readily saturated. The most effective modulators (such as verapamil and cyclosporine) evidently bind the P-gp molecule at sites different from the effluxing binding site.

3.14 Chemotherapy strategies directed at specific oncogenes

The identification of the central role played by the various oncogenes in specific neoplasms is opening up a whole new field of anticancer drug pharmacology. The search is on for novel compounds that will bind and inactivate mutant or overexpressed oncogenes. Mutant p53 is also a potential target as it is known that only one allele in cells need be abnormal for the cell to be functionally p53 negative. Some mutant forms of the p53 protein appear to bind to the normal p53 protein preventing it from functioning.

There is increasing interest in classes of compound that are known collectively as signal transduction inhibitors. Oncogenes such as *ras* and *raf* are components of a complex signalling system that responds to such stimuli as interaction between a receptor on the cell membrance and some growth factor. For the oncogene to 'pass on' its growth-signalling message it may have to undergo some type of chemical change, such as phosphorylation or linking with compounds such as farnesyl alcohol. A number of drugs have been found that appear specifically to inhibit one or other transduction steps, thus potentially stopping cell proliferation.

Another approach that shows considerable promise in experimental systems is the use of antisense oligonucleotides. These are short segments of DNA nucleotides (8 to 20 bases in length) that are coded opposite to a key sequence in the messenger RNA. The antisense DNA will have the same sequence as a key region in the coding strand of the cellular DNA and, therefore, will be complementary to the 'sense' strand of messenger RNA. The antisense nucleotide molecule will bind to the RNA, thus inhibiting protein synthesis. The longer the nucleic acid segment the more specific will be the binding to the desired region in the messenger RNA. If the oligonucleotide is too small then the binding will be largely nonspecific and the ability to shut down protein synthesis selectively will be lost. Conversely, an oligonucleotide of excessive length will present great problems in terms of delivery to the cell and intracellular transport. Antisense RNA can be utilized but may present problems with respect to synthesis and stability. Ribozymes are a type of RNA with enzymatic activity that will cleave specific messenger RNA, thus halting protein synthesis; they have potential as antisense therapeutic agents. If the antisense inhibition is sustained for a sufficient period of time, the cells may cease proliferating or spontaneously undergo apoptosis. As well, they may become very sensitive to chemotherapeutic action. Antisense *bcl-2* has been shown to be very effective in producing these effects *in vitro* with cells that are overexpressing the *bcl-2* protein. A technical problem yet to be overcome satisfactorily is getting the nucleotides to the tumour *in vivo*. The free antisense compound is quickly degraded by nucleases in the serum. The antisense nucleic acid must be protected by some type of encapsulation or chemical modification, or possibly introduced into the tumour cells by a virus vector. There are more and more reports in the literature indicating that antisense treatments directed at a large variety of oncogenes are capable of inhibiting a great many types of cancer cell *in vitro*. There have been demonstrations in some animal studies that antisense therapy is capable of eradicating certain transplanted tumours, and clinical trials utilizing anti-*ras* and anti-*bcl-2* are being undertaken.

It seems that the problem of tumour heterogeneity will still be present even with therapeutic agents as highly specific as antisense nucleotides. Antisense-resistant cells have been seen that have increased intracellular nuclease activity, thus breaking down the oligonucleotides before they can inhibit DNA transcription. Nonetheless, it seems very probable that the availability of such types of drug should significantly augment our capacity to treat malignancy. In theory, they could represent the ideal treatment strategy, inhibiting the fundamental molecular processes in the cancer cell. It is not clear at this point whether antisense RNA or DNA would be therapeutically superior. It is even conceivable that combinations of both with multiple oligonucleotide species of each type, directed at the commonest mutation sites, might be required.

3.15   Androgens and oestrogens

Two of the commonest types of human malignancy (breast carcinoma and prostate carcinoma) have been recognized since the 1940s as being sensitive to alterations in the level of oestrogenic and androgenic steroids. Dramatic regression of advanced tumours can be seen when surgical castration is performed or when the hormone effect is blocked at the cellular level. Just as these tumours can respond to exogenously administered sex steroids by increasing their growth rate, withdrawal or blockade of the growth-stimulating hormone can result in very rapid and extensive tumour cell destruction.

Although many of the steps in the process of hormone-associated tumour regression remain to be elucidated, it is now recognized that the basic cell destruction phenomenon is produced through activation of the apoptosis system within the cell. The main function of the growth-stimulating steroids is to stop apoptosis from occurring and to facilitate continuous passage of the cells through the division cycle. This amounts to favouring cell self-renewal over differentiation. In normal cells, regulatory feedback systems operate to maintain the stem cell compartment within defined boundaries and to ensure that a requisite number of cells enter the differentiation pathway. With normal prostate during hormone withdrawal, most of the differentiated cells undergo apoptosis and most of the tissue stem cells enter a quiescent state. In malignancy, however, the balance between renewal and differentiation/apoptosis is altered and there is a progressive expansion in the number of tumour stem cells.

At the time of first presentation, a great majority (>90%) of prostate cancers and a considerable proportion of breast cancer (approximately 50%) retain sufficient of the normal signal pathways that they will undergo apoptosis when the hormonal stimulus is withdrawn or blocked by antihormones. The nature of the response differs from the usual chemotherapy-induced response in that it is said to follow zero-order kinetics. That is, there is not a linear dose response effect but rather once the functional level of stimulatory hormone falls below a threshold then the process of cell lysis proceeds to completion.

In the case of surgical castration, the effect is clinically often very dramatic and may persist for many months or longer. In a sense this type of apoptosis-induced therapy represents a paradigm of what really effective cancer treatment should be. Nearly all signs of disease may disappear and the cost in toxicity (compared with chemotherapy) is minimal. The problem of course is that not all patients respond and the effect is not permanent. Sooner or later the cancer recurs (even when the patient is maintained on antihormonal therapy). Resistance to all types of hormone manipulation eventually develops, though the tumour may still respond to cytotoxic chemotherapy. The question is whether the hormone refractory state is analogous in any way to the selection of drug-resistant mutants by chemotherapy.

Studies carried out on a number of cell lines that have been derived from hormone-sensitive cells demonstrate a variety of molecular changes associated with the hormone-resistant state. These include mutations in genes coding for hormone receptors and upregulation of certain oncogenes that are known to block apoptosis (*bcl-2*) as well as mutations in p53. That there are a number of genetic changes that lead to hormone resistance is beyond question; the issue is whether they have occurred spontaneously or whether they have been specifically induced by the state of hormone deprivation.

Fluctuation tests to determine whether the hormone-resistant pheno-type is spontaneous or induced have rarely been done. In 1982 Isaacs found the appearance of hormone-resistant prostate carcinoma in rats consistent with a spontaneous origin, but the sample size used in the experiments was small and the results appear not to have been repeated.

Whether the hormone resistance is induced or not, it appears that it is associated with specific genetic changes and that the hormonal milieu favours selection of phenotypes that are capable of autonomous growth. That the environment may operate to influence the rate of appearance of the mutants is suggested by the studies of Noble (1982) and Bruchovsky (1992) which demonstrated that intermittent hormone blockade delays the ultimate development of hormone resistance.

(Hormone-dependent tumours that lose their sensitivity to hormone withdrawal are described as *autonomous.*)

An important question is whether the appropriate use of drugs and hormones together can produce a greater effect then either modality alone or given sequentially. One manoeuvre that has been tried is to stimulate the tumour to growth intentionally by providing the appropriate stimulatory sex hormone and then to utilize chemotherapy. The assumption here is that it is the kinetic state of the tumour cells that will be most important in dictating response. By driving the proliferative state maximally, the growth fraction[†] of the tumour will increase and the generation time of component cells will be reduced. The thinking has been that this will render the tumour population more drug sensitive, reasoning by analogy with the studies of Bruce and coworkers with respect to the sensitivity of resting versus proliferating bone marrow cells (Chapter 2).

Clinical trials of this strategy have been attempted in both breast and prostate cancer, but with basically negative results. In a few cases, serious clinical problems developed because of tumour stimulation without any associated chemotherapy benefit. In hindsight it is perhaps apparent as to why the strategy has not been successful. If the tumour cells were genetically resistant to chemotherapy (for example by expressing P-gp) then increased growth rate would not render them susceptible to chemotherapy. In addition, the nature of the growth stimulation provided by the hormones is probably the wrong kind for generating drug sensitivity. Stimulation by sexual steroids appears to act primarily by blocking apoptosis rather then providing an independent growth signal. This would actually work against a chemotherapy effect even if the tumour cells were potentially more sensitive by virtue of rapid growth kinetics.

Hormonal suppressive therapy could act indirectly to reduce the problem of drug resistance simply on the basis of general reduction in tumour mass. If there are any drug-resistant mutants that are still susceptible to hormone-associated apoptosis then this would be expected to contribute to cytotoxic therapy effectiveness.

[†] Growth fraction is the proportion of tumour cells that are proliferating (i.e. synthesizing DNA) relative to the entire tumour population. Experimental mouse leukaemias have growth fractions of nearly 100% whereas many clinical solid tumours have estimated growth fraction < 10%. The percentage of proliferating cells is *not* equivalent to the percentage of stem cells within the tumour, which will typically be much smaller than the growth fractions.

3.16   Glucocorticoids

Another very important class of antitumour steroid hormones is the family of glucocorticoid compounds (hydrocortisone plus a large number of potent synthetic analogues). The glucocorticoids mediate a wide range of physiological functions including salt, water, glucose and protein metabolism as well as modulating a variety of immune responses. Glucocorticoids play a key role in the development of normal lymphoid cells by initiating apoptosis in those lymphoid cells that are surplus to physiological requirements. It is this property that makes the glucocorticoids useful in the treatment of immunological disorders or as immune suppressants in organ transplantation.

A number of malignancies of the lymphoid system retain their sensitivity to glucocortcoid-induced apoptosis. The glucocorticoids are useful therapeutic agents in treating a variety of lymphoid-derived tumours (lymphoblastic leukaemia, various categories of non-Hodgkin's lymphoma, Hodgkin's disease, multiple myeloma, etc.). The apoptosis induced by glucocorticoids in lymphoid tissues is not dependent on normal p53 function, a circumstance which probably contributes significantly to the broad antilymphoma effect seen with glucocorticoids.

Acquired resistance to glucocorticoids appears to conform closely to the pattern seen with classical drug resistance mechanisms. A common molecular alteration seen in glucocorticoid resistance involves mutations in the glucocorticoid receptors on the cell surface. Studies have suggested that the mutation rate to glucocorticoid resistance in a variety of lymphoid cell lines is in the order of 10^{-5} to 10^{-10}.

The mechanism of cell lysis induced by the glucocorticoids appears to be different from that seen with the androgenic and oestrogenic steroids and to be confined to tumours of lymphoid origin. However, their ability to induce rapid tumour lysis without any associated haematological suppression makes the glucocorticoids invaluable antitumour agents.

3.17   Radiation effects and drug resistance

At a fundamental level there appears to be a number of similarities between cytotoxic chemotherapy and ionizing radiation. Radiation, like chemotherapy, produces a log–linear dose response effect on all the cells that are capable of undergoing proliferation. It is now recognized that a major component of radiation-induced cell killing involves the induction of apoptosis through both the p53-dependent and p53-independent pathways. Tumour cells that are homozygous negative for p53 function exhibit increased radiation resistance compared with similar tumours that are p53 positive.

An important early event in radiation effect is activation of a group of coordinately acting genes collectively designated as 'early response' genes. These genes are induced in the early stages of repair of radiation-induced damage. If the amount of damage exceeds the capacity of the repair system then apoptosis is induced. This would certainly suggest that there is a major genetic element in radiation sensitivity and resistance in addition to the influence of local tissue environmental factors (oxygen tension, pH, vascularity) that have been emphasized. It is surprising, therefore, that it has proved difficult to demonstrate any selection effect for radiation resistance by means of repeat radiation exposure. There have been a few experiments that suggest that a selection phenomenon can occur (Courtney, 1965), but some of these have involved radiation environments (chronic exposure to deuterated water) quite different from those involved in clinical and experimental radiotherapy. Simplistically, one might have expected courses of radiation to select for p53 null cells from within a heterogeneous population, but this has not been reported. Different types of tumour, as well as different individual patients, show wide ranges in intrinsic radiation sensitivity, but it has been difficult to demonstrate selection for radioresistant subtypes. Likewise, chemotherapy does not appear to select for radioresistant mutants even while selecting for cells that have enhanced DNA repair capacity.

In the late 1980s, some experimenters reported finding what appear to be true radioresistant variants that were selected for radiation resistance out of a radiosensitive population. The process to produce these variants was basically similar to that which has been employed in classical chemotherapy experiments. A critical factor in these radiation studies was the use by the experimenters of radiation dosages and schedules that were similar to those employed clinically. That is, they utilized exposures of 2 Gy (gray) per radiation fraction. Both stable and unstable variants were cloned from the initial cell population and their relative radioresistance confirmed by the appropriate colony-forming assays. The degree of radioresistance by these criteria tended to be considerably less than that produced by selection for drug-resistant variants but, nevertheless, it would appear to be sufficient to cause major problems with respect to treatment outcome. The molecular basis for this radioresistance is uncertain but it was associated with a diminished ability of the cells to undergo apoptosis following radiation exposure. Identification of the molecular changes associated with this type of radioresistance could be a very significant finding leading as it might to improved approaches for producing clinical radiosensitization.

Hill has demonstrated that radiation doses in the range used therapeutically generate a broad range of drug-resistant mutants and at relatively high rates. This phenomenon is consistent with what has been commonly observed clinically, namely that cancers that recur in a radiated field are much less chemosensitive than similar tumours that have not received prior radiation.

That radiation may result in many drug-resistant mutations is not surprising given the known mutagenic effect of high-energy X-rays. In radiobiology the 'G' value is the number of events (e.g. damaged molecules) per 100 eV (electron volts) of absorbed energy. One rad (0.01 Gy) of radiation delivers an amount of energy equal to 100 erg/g tissue, which equals 6.2×10^{13} eV/g. Typical G values are 0.01 to 1 for *each* type of DNA damage (and there are a large number of different types, including single-strand breaks, double-strand breaks, cross-linking, base denaturation, etc.). A typical radiotherapeutic regimen of 60 Gy (6000 rad) will deliver 3.7×10^{17} eV to each gram of tissue. A 100 g tumour will have 10^{10} cells and will contain approximately 100 mg DNA. This means there will be 10^{12} to 10^{14} instances of *any* type of DNA damage in a 100 g tumour. Many of the cells in the tumour will be killed, but any surviving cell will have sustained a heavy load of damaged DNA. Moreover, the damage will not be distributed evenly per cell but will follow a Poisson distribution with some cells receiving considerably more than the average number of DNA lesions.

It is apparent that any residual cell population in radiation-treated tumours will contain a large reservoir of potentially mutated cells. In this sense, radiation is decidedly nonneutral in its effect. Any cells that are not killed will be a great risk for undergoing further mutations, at least some of which might be expected to confer drug resistance. This effect would argue for the use of chemotherapy *prior* to or during radiation in circumstances where this is feasible. This may be the optimal time for maximum chemotherapeutic effect and, as well, would 'down size' the tumour mass, rendering it more likely to be eradicated by the radiation.

3.18   Summary and conclusions

We have reviewed briefly some of the general types of molecular change that are associated with resistance of the antitumour drugs. The enormous capacity for cancer cells to express resistance to large numbers of cytotoxic agents is related to the fact that cells have evolved very efficient mechanisms for protecting themselves from various types of cellular damage. As well, many anticancer agents utilize normal metabolic pathways for part of their action and efficient alternative pathways may exist that can be expressed by drug-resistant cells.

It appears that many, perhaps all, anticancer drugs exert their effect through a final common mechanism, that of programmed cell death or apoptosis. It may be *because* the anticancer drugs access this pathway that they are useful as antitumour agents with a good therapeutic index. Nonspecific cell poisons such as cyanide or azide do not appear to have an exploitable therapeutic index for malignant versus normal cells.

The loss of function such as that seen with p53 mutation, while on the one hand contributing to drug resistance, may be, or the other, a source of exploitable weakness in the cancer cell. By continuously going through the cell cycle and not, as it were, stopping to repair damage, the cancer cell may be rendered vulnerable to certain types of chemotherapy strategy, such as protracted exposure to low levels of certain antineoplastic agents (e.g. 5-FU, ara-C, etoposide). It will be recalled that in the Bruce experiments described in Chapter 2 it was because the lymphoma cells were continuously in cycle that they were especially vulnerable to chemotherapeutic effects.

References

Courtenay, V.D. (1965). The response to continuous irradiation of the mouse lymphoma L51784 grown *in vitro. Int. J. Radiat. Biol.*, 9: 581–592.

Eigen, M. (1992). *Steps Towards Life*. Oxford University Press, Oxford.

Isaacs, J.T. (1982). Cellular factors in the development of resistance to hormonal therapy. In *Drug and Hormone Resistance in Neoplasia*, Vol. I, ed. J.H. Goldie and N. Bruchovsky, pp. 139–156. CRC Press, Boca Raton, FL.

Juliano, R.L. and Ling, V. (1976). A surface glycoprotein modulating drug permeability in Chinese hamster ovary cell mutants. *Biochim. Biophys. Acta*, 455: 152–159.

Lowe, S.W., Ruley, H.E., Jacks, T. *et al.* (1993). p53 dependent apoptosis mod-
ulates the cytotoxicity of anticancer agents. *Cell*, 74: 957–967.

Tsuro, T. (1983). Reversal of acquired resistance to vinca alkaloids and anthra-
cycline antibiotics. *Cancer Treat. Rep.*, 67: 889–894.

Further reading

Altman, K.I., Gerber, G.B. and Okada, S. (1970). *Radiation Biochemistry*, Vol. 1,
pp. 52–56. Academic Press, London.

Bally, M.B., Hope, M.J., Meyer, L. *et al.* (1988). Novel procedures for generating
and loading liposomal systems. Liposomes in drug carriers. *Science 1988;
Recent Trends and Progress*, ed. G. Gregorladis, pp. 841–853. Wiley, New
York.

Berchem, G., Bosseler, M., Sugars, L. *et al.* (1995). Androgens induce resistance
to *bcl-2*-mediated apoptosis in LNCaP prostate cancer cells. *Cancer Res.*, 55:
735–738.

Bradley, G., Juranka, P.F. and Ling, V. (1988). Mechanism of multidrug resistance. *Biochim. Biophys. Acta*, 948: 87–128.

Chabner, B.A. (ed.) (1982). *Pharmacologic Principles of Cancer Treatments.*
Saunders, Philadelphia, PA.

Cole, S.P.C., Bhardway, G., Gerbach, J.H. *et al.* (1992). Overexpression of a
transporter gene in a multidrug resistant human lung cancer cell line.
Science, 258: 1650–1654.

Colombel, M. Olsson, C., Ng, P. and Buttyan, R. (1992). Hormone-regulated
apoptosis results from reentry of differentiated prostate cells onto a defective
cell cycle. *Cancer Res.*, 52: 4313–4319.

Crone, T.M., Goodtzova, K., Edara, S. *et al.* (1994). Mutations in human O^6-
alkylguanine–DNA alkyltransferase imparting resistance to O^6-benzylguanine.
Cancer Res., 54: 6221–6227.

Croop, J.M. (1994). P-glycoprotein structure and homologous evolution. In
Multiple Drug Resistance and Cancer, ed. M. Clynes, pp. 1–32. Kluwer
Academic, Norwell, MA.

DeVita, V.T. Jr (1993). Principles of chemotherapy in cancer. In *Principles and
Practice of Oncology*, ed. R. Baserga, V.T. DeVita, S.A. Hellman, and S.A.
Rosenberg, pp. 276–292. Lippincott, Philadelphia, PA.

Erickson, L.C. (1991). The role of O-6 methylguanine DNA methyltransferase
(MGMT) in drug resistance and strategies for its inhibition. *Cancer Biol.*, 2:
257–265.

Evans, R.M., Laskin, J.D. and Hakala, M.T. (1980). Assessment of growth limiting
events caused by 5-fluorouracil in mouse cells and in human cells. *Cancer
Res.*, 40: 4112–4113.

Fan, S., El-Deiry, W.S., Bae, I. *et al.* (1994). p53 gene mutations are associated with decreased sensitivity of human lymphoma cells to DNA damaging agents. *Cancer Res.*, 54: 5824–5830.

Friedberg, E.C. (1984). *DNA Repair.* Francis, New York.

Fujimori, A., Harker, W.G., Kohlhagen, G. *et al.* (1995). Mutation at the catalytic site of topoisomerase I in CEM/C2, a human leukemia cell line resistant to camptothecin. *Cancer Res.*, 55: 1339–1346.

Goldenberg, G.T. and Begleiter, B. (1980). Membrane transport of alkylating agents. *Pharmacol. Ther.*, 8: 237–274.

Goldman, I.D. (1971). The characteristics of the membrane transport of amethopterin and the naturally occurring folates. *Ann. NY Acad. Sci.*, 186: 400–422.

Goldman, I.D. (1982). Pharmacokinetics of antineoplastic agents at the cellular level. In *Pharmacologic Principles of Cancer Treatment*, ed. B.A. Chabner. Saunders, Philadelphia, PA.

Graham, F.L. and Whitmore, G.F. (1970). Studies in mouse L-cells on the incorporation of 1-β-D-arabinofuranosylcytosine into DNA and on the inhibition of DNA polymerase by 1-β-D-arabinofuranosylcytosine-5-triphosphate. *Cancer Res.*, 30: 2636–2644.

Graham II, M., Krett, N., Miller, L. *et al.* (1990). T47D$_{co}$ cells, genetically unstable and containing estrogen receptor mutations, are a model for the progression of breast cancers to hormone resistance. *Cancer Res.*, 50: 6208–6217.

Greenblatt, M.S., Bennett, W.P., Hollstein, M. *et al.* (1994). Mutations in the *p53* tumour suppressor gene: clues to cancer etiology and molecular pathogenesis. *Cancer Res.*, 54: 4855–4878.

Hill, B.T. (1993). Differing patterns of cross resistance from exposure to specific anti-tumour drugs and radiation *in vitro. Cytotechnology*, 12: 265–288.

Huet-Minkowski, M., Gasson, J.C. and Bourgeois, S. (1982). Glucocorticoid resistance in lymphoid cell lines. In *Drug and Hormone Resistance in Neoplasia*, Vol. I, ed. J.H. Goldie and N. Bruchovsky, pp. 79–94. CRC Press, Boca Raton, FL.

Kamada, S., Shimono, A., Shinto, Y. *et al.* (1995). *bcl-2* deficiency in mice leads to pleiotropic abnormalities: accelerated lymphoid cell death in thymus and spleen, polycystic kidney, hair hypopigmentation, and distorted small intestine. *Cancer Res.*, 55: 354–359.

Kellen, J.A. *et al.* (1994). *Reversal of Multi-Drug Resistance. In Cancer 1994*, CRC Press, Boca Raton, FL.

Kitada, S., Takayama, S., de Riel, K. *et al.* (1994). Reversal of chemoresistance of lymphoma cells by antisense-mediated reduction of *bcl-2* gene expression. *Antisense Res. Dev.*, 4: 71–79.

Kobayashi, H., Man, S., Graham, C.H. *et al.* (1993). Acquired multicellular-mediated resistance to alkylating agents in cancer. *Proc. Natl. Acad. Sci. USA*, 90: 3294–3298.

Lin, L.F. and Wang, J.C. (1991). Biochemistry of DNA topoisomerases and their poisons. In *DNA Topoisomerases in Cancer*, ed. M. Potmeril, K.W. Kohn *et al.*, pp. 13–22. Oxford University Press, Oxford.

Ling, V. and Thompson, L.H. (1974). Reduced permeability in CHO cells as a mechanism of resistance to colchicine. *J. Cell. Physiol.*, 83: 103–110.

Looney, W.E. and Hopkins, H.A. (1993). Experimental and clinical rationale for alternating chemotherapy and radiotherapy in human cancer management in chemoradiation. In *Ingegrated Approach to Cancer Treatment*, ed. M.J. John, M.S. Flam, S.S. Leghy and T.L. Phillips, pp. 217–252. Yen and Fetiger, Philadelphia, PA.

Martin, S.J. and Green, D.R. (1995). Apoptosis and cancer: the failure of controls on cell death and cell survival. *Article Rev. Oncol./Hematol.*, 18: 137–153.

Moalli, P. and Rosen, S. (1994). Glucocorticoid receptors and resistance to glucocorticoids in hematologic malignancies. *Leukemia and Lymphoma*, 15: 363–374.

Moscow, J.A. and Dixon, K.H. (1994). Glutathione-related enzymes, glutathione and multi-drug resistance. In *Multiple Drug Resistance in Cancer*, ed. M. Clynes, M., pp. 155–170. Kluwer Academic, Norvell, MA.

Mukhopadhyay, T. and Roth, J. (1995). Antisense Therapy for Cancer. *Cancer J.*, 1: 233–242.

Noble, R.L. (1982). Tumour progression endocrine regulation and control. In *Drug and Hormone Resistance in Neoplasia*; Vol. I, ed. J.H. Goldie and N. Bruchovsky, pp. 157–183. CRC Press, Boca Raton, FL.

Nooter, K., Boersma, A., Oostrum, R. *et al.* (1995). Constitutive expression of the c-H-*ras* oncogene inhibits doxorubicin-induced apoptosis and promotes cell survival in a rhabdomyosarcoma cell line. *Br. J. Cancer*, 71: 556–561.

Perry, M.C. (ed.) (1992). *The Chemotherapy Source Book*. Williams & Wilkins, Baltimore, MD.

Pierga, J.Y. and Magdelenat, H. (1994). Applications of antisense oligonucleotides in oncology. *Cell. Mol. Biol.*, 40: 237–261.

Powell, S.N. and Abraham, E.H. (1993). The biology of radiation resistance: simularities, differences and interactions with drug resistance. *Cytotechnology*, 12: 325–345.

Reed, J. (1995). *BCL-2*: prevention of apoptosis as a mechanism of drug resistance. *Hematol./Oncol. Clinics N. Am.*, 9: 451–473.

Reichard, P., Skold, O., Klein, G. *et al.* (1962). Studies on resistance against 5-fluorouracil 1. Enzymes of the uracil pathway during development of resistance. *Cancer Res.*, 22: 235–243.

Roberts, J.J., Brent, T.P. and Crathorn, A.R. (1971). Evidence for the inactivation and repair of the mammalian DNA template after alkylations by mustard gas and half mustard gas. *Eur. J. Cancer*, 7: 515–421.

Russel, J., Wheldon, T.E. and Stanton, P. (1995). A radio-resistant variant derived from a human neuroblastoma cell line is less prone to radiation-induced apoptosis. *Cancer Rev.*, 4915–4921.

Sancur, A. and Sancur, G.B. (1988). DNA repair enzymes. *Annu. Rev. Biochem.*, 57: 29–67.

Segal-Bendirdjian, E. and Jacquemin-Sablon, A. (1995). Cisplatin resistance in a murine leukemia cell line is associated with a defective apoptotic process. *Exp. Cell Res.*, 218: 201–212.

Sinha, B., Yamazaki, H., Eliot, H. *et al.* (1995). Relationships between proto-oncogene expression and apoptosis induced by anticancer drugs in human prostate tumour cells. *Biochim. Biophys. Acta*, 1270: 12–18.

Strasser-Wozak, E., Hattmannstorfer, R., Hala, M. *et al.* (1995). Splice site mutation in the glucocorticoid receptor gene causes resistance in glucocorticoid-induced apoptosis in a human acute leukemic cell line. *Cancer Res.*, 55: 348–353.

Taverna, P., Hansson, J., Scanlon, K.J. *et al.* (1994). Gene expression in X-irradiated human tumour cell lines expressing cisplatin resistance and altered DNA repair capacity. *Carcinogenesis*, 15: 2053–2056.

Thompson, C.B. (1995). Apoptosis in the pathogenesis and treatment of disease. *Science*, 267: 1456–1462.

Wattel, E., Preudhomme, C., Hecquet, B. *et al.* (1994). *p53* mutations are associated with resistance to chemotherapy and short survival in hematologic malignancies. *Blood*, 84: 3148–3157.

Weichselbaum, R.R., Beckett, M.A., Schwartz, J.L. *et al.* (1988). Radioresistant tumor cells are present in head and neck carcinomas that recur after radiotherapy. *Int. J. Radiat. Oncol. Biol. Phys.*, 15: 575–579.

Xia, F., Wang, X., Wang, Y. *et al.* (1995). Altered *p53* status correlates with differences in sensitivity to radiation-induced mutation and apoptosis in two closely related human lymphoblast lines. *Cancer Res.*, 55: 12–15.

Yaes, R.J. (1989). Tumour heterogeneity, tumour size and radio-resistance. *Int. J. Radiat. Oncol. Physics*, 17: 993–1005.

Yarosh, D.B., Foote, R.S., Mitra, S. *et al.* (1983). Repair of O^6-methylguanine in DNA by demethylation is lacking in MER minus human tumour cell strains. *Carcinogenesis*, 4: 199–205.

4

Quantitative descriptions of the origins of drug resistance

4.1 Introduction

In this chapter we will begin to discuss resistance in quantitative terms. Chapter 3 contained a discussion of the molecular and cellular processes by which resistance arises; this will not be addressed here. The purpose here is to describe the development of resistance using formulae so that predictions regarding the distribution and onset of resistance can be made. The beautiful thing about formulae is that they tell you everything and nothing about the nature of a system. Everything, in that a correct complete formulae tells you exactly how the process will evolve and what affects it. Nothing, in that identical formulae may apply to quite different mechanisms of effect so that it is not possible, in general, to discern the 'how' from the structure of an equation. Quite different mechanisms of resistance may (or may not) have formulae describing their development that are functionally the same. Formulae describing a system may be derived, in general, in two ways.

One method is to build a model for the system of interest using known characteristics of the system. As an example consider building a model to describe the length of a steel spring. Hook's law indicates that the extension of a steel spring is proportional to the force applied to it. Also, steel expands upon heating so that we would expect the length to depend upon the ambient temperature. Other physical mechanisms with known modes of action may be postulated and piece by piece a model for the system constructed. Using known mathematical equations that describe each of these processes a composite set of equations for the whole system may be developed and then solved to provide formulae that relate the outcome of interest (the length of the spring) to the factors which influence it (force, temperature, etc.). We will term this a theoretical model-building approach.

The second approach is to utilize directly observations on the system of interest and on factors thought to affect it. In cases where the factors thought to affect the outcome can be directly manipulated, this represents the classical experimental approach. A series of experiments would be carried out to measure the length of the spring at different forces, temperatures, etc. In many situations, direct manipulation of factors is not possible (e.g. astronomy) and one makes measurement of the outcome at times or places where the factors are different. Having gained these data, graphical or statistical techniques are used to determine the nature of the formula that relates the factors to the outcome. One may term this an empirical model-building approach.

In the development which follows, we will use a theoretical model building approach, using processes identified in experimental systems, to build a model for the effect of chemotherapy on clinical cancer.

Before continuing it is necessary to define some terms so that there is no confusion later. A mathematical or statistical model represents a description, using formulae, of the behaviour of a process. A parameter in a model represents a constant that relates the dependence of the outcome of interest (development or resistance, say) to some factors which influence it. Therefore, in the example of Hook's law, the extension, E, of the spring is related to the stretching force, F, by

$$E = kF. \tag{4.1}$$

The constant of proportionality, k, is a parameter and Equation 4.1 is a model for the extension, E, of a spring subject to a stretching force, F. What we now wish to develop is a model that relates the development of resistance to factors likely to affect it. In order to do so we will spend a section discussing the development of mathematical and probabilistic models, and how they may be manipulated to provide different formulations of the same process.

4.2 Development of mathematical models of biological systems

As described above, models of systems may be built from a synthesis of statements about the way individual factors influence outcome or from an empirical *fit* of relationships via graphical or statistical methods. Having derived a model it may be mathematically manipulated to alter its appearance. Such alterations may be from an aesthetic viewpoint or from a desire to conform to some standard mode of presentation. More seriously though, one expression may provide more insight into the behaviour of the system or permit simpler generalization to more complex systems. Consider Hook's law. We can rewrite this by finding the change in extension brought about by an increase in the stretching force. If E_1 is the extension when force F_1 is applied and E_2 is the (increased) extension when (a greater) force F_2 is applied then

$$E_1 = kF_1$$
$$E_2 = kF_2$$

By subtracting the second equation from the first we obtain,

$$E_2 - E_1 = k(F_2 - F_1).$$

Now it is common mathematic notation to designate a change in something by the Greek letter Δ. Therefore, we can rewrite Hook's model for the extension of a spring as

$$\Delta E = k\Delta F,$$

the increase in extension, ΔE, is proportional to the increase in stretching force, ΔF. Again manipulating this a little further we have

$$\frac{\Delta E}{\Delta F} = k.$$

The ratio of increased extension to increased force is a constant. Finally, if we refer to calculus we may take the limiting process, where we consider smaller and smaller increases in the applied force F so that we obtain the differential equation

$$\frac{dE}{dF} = k.$$

This equation says that the rate of change of E as F changes is a constant. In what follows in the discussion of resistance, we will wish to manipulate relationships to have a different mathematical form so that they may be more easily incorporated into a comprehensive model of drug resistance.

We wish to utilize some measure of resistance in a population of cells and relate it to factors thought to influence it. As was suggested in Chapter 1, the most obvious measure of resistance in a population of cells is the number of cells that are resistant. When resistance is thought of as relative this reduces to the number of cells that are 'more' resistant.

Depending on the biochemical mechanism that confers resistance, the relative scale may be a continuum (e.g. gene amplification) or may only contain two states (presence or absence of a specific enzyme). Measures other than the number of resistant cells can be used to characterize a cell population. For example, we could use the presence or absence or cells resistant to a particular drug concentration, or the maximum concentration to which one or more cells are resistant. Having chosen the number of resistant cells we will now give it a symbolic representation, R. Thus we wish to model the way in which R depends on factors thought to influence it. The same problem was faced in the 1930s by researchers exploring the phenomenon of resistance in bacterial populations to antibiotics or viral infection. We will discuss the questions that these researchers posed and present the analyses they developed to answer those questions.

4.3 Quantitative theories for the development of resistance by bacteria to viral infection

As the number of active antibiotics increased the importance of the phenomenon of resistance grew correspondingly. Attempts to study the phenomenon were plagued with apparent technical problems of wildly fluctuating results leading to inconsistency of interpretation. However, there was a common pattern, exposure of bacterial cells to an antibiotic resulted in the rapid death of the vast majority of cells. If the total population exposed was below some critical number, the whole population was eliminated. If the population size exceeded this threshold then a subpopulation would survive. If the population was at, or close to, the threshold, then a surviving population sometimes existed and sometimes did not. Further exposure of the surviving cells to repeat application of the drug did not result in extinction of the population and indeed, in some cases, the surviving cells appeared to replicate as well in the drug-containing environment as the parent cells had functioned in the drug-free environment.

The consistency of the above pattern in different bacteria and for resistance to different agents convinced investigators at that time that they were witnessing phenomena that had a similar process of causation. However, there was considerable uncertainty as to its origin. The sustained nature of the change in sensitivity suggested that this was a characteristic which could be transmitted to cellular progeny. Its permanence, after removal of the challenge, suggested that this characteristic was now part of the cell line. These observations taken together implied a relationship to the genetic structure of the cell. Hence it became widely believed that the resistance of some cells was a result of genetic differences between them and these other cells which succumbed to the agent. Accepting that genetic differences were the determinants of resistance, how did these differences arise? It did not take long for a number of theories to be proposed as to how such events occurred. These soon became focused on two main concepts.

One concept, frequently referred to as *Lamarkian* in the literature of the time, hypothesized an interaction between drug (or virus) and the cell whereby the cell gained the ability to resist the action of the agent. The exact mechanism for this 'transfer or acquisition of information' was not specified. However, several mechanisms may exist for different drugs so that a unique specification was not possible, especially given the limits of the technology of the time. The information acquired somehow altered the genetic structure of the cell and was passed along to future generations. In order that not all cells become resistant it was further hypothesized that the process was imperfect, with only a fraction of cells acquiring resistance. The reason for this 'partial acquisition' was hypothesized to competition between this process and the killing effect of the drug or virus. We will refer to this as the *directed mutation (induction) model.* (The term 'directed mutation' is now more often used to denote this process; it implies that the environmental substance *specifically* induces or directs the mutational change in the cell.) The second hypothesis, which could be termed *Darwinian*, was that genetic alterations were randomly occurring all the time. A small fraction of these alterations confer resistance in a cell to a particular agent. The effect of subsequent drug application is to select out the resistant cells and destroy those which are sensitive. This leaves the small fraction that are resistant, which then repopulate the tumour. We will refer to the second model as a *random mutation (selection) model.* Figure 4.1 schematically illustrates these two hypotheses in a growing cell population.

Of course there is nothing about either the Lamarkian or the Darwinian process which excludes the presence of the other. Both processes may take place. In different cases one or the other may dominate. Any 'proof' of the existence of one of these processes in a particular example does not imply the nonexistence of the other or indicate what happens in general. However, the proven existence of one process,

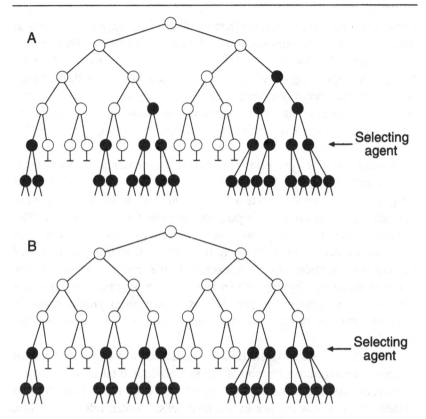

Fig. 4.1. Schemes A and B indicate the growth of a hypothetical system from a single cell through four synchronized divisions to a population of 16 cells. In A, resistance (indicated by solid circles) is assumed to arise via a random mutation process whereas in B it is assumed to arise via a directed process. In both A and B the number of resistant cells after four divisions is the same and occur in the same pedigree. The frequency of resistance is made artificially high to permit simple depiction. In A, the resistant cells exist prior to the application of the selecting agent (drug) whereas in B the application causes the conversion of some existing sensitive cells to a state of resistance.

without contrary examples, will tend to make us believe that this process holds exclusively. In any situation where both processes exist they may occur at different frequencies so that only the more common one is demonstrable.

The first investigator to present evidence for pre-existing variation in bacterial populations was Burnett in 1929. Individual colonies of salmonellae may show either a 'rough' or 'smooth' appearance. This in turn is related to the composition of the bacterial capsule. Burnett was able to show that there were differences in sensitivity to lysis by bacteriophage depending on whether the colonies were smooth or rough, suggesting that some inherent genetic property of the bacteria was what was determining their resistance to bacteriophage infection. These observations led Burnett to postulate a Darwinian origin for resistant microbes.

In principle it is very easy to distinguish whether a random mutation process is present. The random mutation hypothesis implies that drug-naive cells grown from a single cell will, if grown to a large enough size, contain a subpopulation of cells that are resistant. The directed mutation model implies that the same population will contain no resistant cells. We assume in both cases that the possibility of starting with a resistant cell is excluded. We can, therefore, decide between these two hypotheses by determining whether resistant cells are present in drug-naive populations grown from single sensitive cells. In order to do this we must first overcome two experimental difficulties.

Firstly, it is necessary to characterize resistance in a way that does not depend on drug administration. The most obvious method is to have a marker, obtained from studies in drug-resistant cells, that is known to be present in such cells but not in sensitive cells. We can refer to this first requirement as specificity. Secondly, it must be possible to measure this marker with great accuracy in large populations of cells, so that if it is present in 1 cell in 10^{12} (say) it can be detected. We may term this quality sensitivity. Practically, the requirements of both sensitivity and specificity represent a formidable challenge even today and were insurmountable in the 1930s.

Therefore, indirect means to address the question of the origin of resistant subtypes were sought. It was not until 1943, with the publication of a paper by Luria and Delbrück, that a solution was forthcoming. Their experimental method, known as the *fluctuation test*, provided a method for discriminating between these two hypotheses. The essence of their approach is a recognition that the two models imply different things about the development of resistance in a growing cell population over time. In order to discuss this experiment we will now review the quantitative implications of the two mutation models and present an introduction to probabilistic modelling.

4.4   Probabilistic descriptions of the models for the development of resistance

Directed mutation model

First consider the directed mutation model. In its simplest form it implies that at administration of the drug a proportion of cells will become resistant. We will refer to this proportion as ρ. Therefore, if N is the number of cells present at the time of drug administration, then the induction model says that the number of resistant cells created, R, will be

$$R = \rho N. \tag{4.2}$$

If, as is often useful, we think of these quantities as being a function of time, then prior to drug administration at time t^* there are no resistant cells. At t^*, ρN resistant cells are created, which then continue to grow according to their kinetics and the environmental conditions. Although useful for describing what will happen on average, Equation 4.2 requires some refinement to be used for predicting the outcome of an individual experiment.

We know that if the number of sensitive cells, N, is small, frequently none will become resistant upon drug application although Equation 4.2 predicts that some number will. Similarly, the number of resistant cells is a whole number, fractions do not exist and Equation 4.2 will only yield integral values for R for certain values of N. This problem arises because a discrete process is being modelled by a continuous mathematical function. A common approach to remedy this is to continue to use the equation and round to the nearest whole number, so that if $\rho N < 0.5$ set $R = 0$, if $0.5 \leq \rho N < 1.5$ set $R = 1$, etc. This is unlikely to cause much of a problem when $\rho N \cong 1000$; however, when $\rho N \cong 0.5$, the difference between $R = 1$ and $R = 0$ is quite considerable. A population with $R = 1$ will survive administration of the drug, a population with $R = 0$ will not. A more suitable approach is to use probability models and to consider the number of resistant cells to follow a probability distribution.

The *probability distribution* of a process is a formula that assigns a number between 0 and 1, the probability, for each *state* a system may occupy. A *state* of a system represents any possible condition the system could be in. When trying to describe the number of resistant cells in a population of N cells there are $N + 1$ possible states representing 0 resistant cells, 1 resistant cell, . . ., N resistant cells. The question is then, how do we specify what is the probability distribution of these states? As above we could select the state which is closest to ρN and set the probability of that state equal to 1. This essentially duplicates the nearest whole number approach described in the preceding paragraph. Another way is to make some further observations (or assumptions) about the behaviour of each cell when exposed to the drug under the induction model. Drawing on our discussion of Hook's law in Section 4.2, we may reformulate Equation 4.2 as the change in the number of resistant cells, ΔR, when extra cells, ΔN, are exposed to the drug, i.e.

$$\Delta R = \rho \Delta N. \tag{4.3}$$

For the particular case when only one extra cell is exposed to the drug ($\Delta N = 1$), we obtain from Equation 4.3 that the number of resistant cells should increase by $\rho (\Delta R = \rho \times 1 = \rho)$. Unfortunately this does not solve the problem as we shall still have some 'pieces' of resistant cells. However, we may use this formulation to develop a probability model. Instead we may think of ρ as the probability that the extra cell exposed to the drug is converted to resistance. In symbols we would write this as

$$P\{\Delta R = 1 | \Delta N = 1\} = \rho :$$

in words, this is the probability that the number of resistant cells increases by unity when one sensitive cell is exposed to the drug. Similarity between the probabilistic and nonprobabilistic approaches can be seen by examining the average increase in the number of resistant cells in the probabilistic model. In general, the average increase is equal to the sum of all possible values of (the increase in the number of resistant cells × the probability that increase will occur). In this case we have only two possibilities: an increase of 1 with a probability of ρ and an increase of 0 with a probability of $1 - \rho$. Therefore, we have:

$$\text{average increase} = 1 \times \rho + 0 \times (1 - \rho) = \rho.$$

If we assume that each cell has the same probability, upon exposure, of developing resistance, ρ, then the average number of cells which develop resistance will be this probability multiplied by the number of cells, N, i.e. ρN. Under these assumptions we reproduce Equation 4.2 as the average number of resistant cells. In order for this formula to hold we must assume that each cell has the same value of ρ, i.e. cells are all equally likely to develop resistance. If we make the further assumption that resistance developing in one cell does not influence the likelihood that resistance will develop in another cell,[†] then the number of resistant cells has a probability distribution known as the binomial distribution. This is the same distribution used for determining the number of heads observed in several coin tosses. In this case ρ is the probability of heads and N is the number of tosses. When ρ is small and N is large the binomial distribution is well approximated by a Poisson distribution with parameter ρN. The formula for the distribution (see also Chapter 2) is given by

$$P\{R = r\} = \frac{(\rho N)^r}{r!} e^{-\rho N}. \tag{4.4}$$

The mean and variance of the distribution is given by

$$\text{mean} = \mu = \rho N,$$
$$\text{variance} = \sigma^2 = \rho N, \tag{4.5}$$

where μ and σ^2 are standard symbols for the mean and variance. The standard deviation $\sigma = \sqrt{(\rho N)}$ and is the square root of the variance; it measures the likely degree of variability of R about its mean, μ. Since the standard deviation is proportional to $\sqrt{N}$, the absolute variability of the number of resistant cells increases as the number of sensitive cells exposed to the drug increases. The relative variation, as measured by the ratio of the standard deviation to the mean,

$$\frac{\sigma}{\mu} = \frac{1}{\sqrt{\rho N}},$$

decreases as the mean increases so that fluctuations around the mean become proportionately smaller. We can summarize our analysis to this point by saying that when the expected number of resistant cells is large consideration of the actual distribution will provide little extra information. When the expected number is small consideration of the distribution is essential.

The probability that there are no resistant cells, $R = 0$, is given by substituting $r = 0$ into Equation 4.4 to give

---

[†] This concept is referred to as *independence*. In fact it is because in the random mutation model the probability of a cell being resistant is altered by the observation that another cell is resistant (*nonindependence*) that Luria and Delbrück were able to develop the fluctuation test.

$$P\{R = r\} = e^{-\rho N}. \tag{4.6}$$

This relationship will be used later.

Now if the Poisson distribution gives the number of resistant cells after application of the drug, what is the number at some later point? Obviously this will depend on the number present after drug administration and the kinetics of resistant cell growth. For bacterial populations growing in the conditions of these experiments, exponential growth is a reasonable assumption. If we assume that the exponential growth is perfectly regular and the cells have common division time τ, then each cell grows to size $2^{t/\tau}$ in an interval of time of length t. If we then carry through the calculations involved we find that the mean number of resistant cells at time t, after exposure to the drug is

$$\text{mean} = \rho N 2^{t/\tau},$$

with $\hspace{8cm}$ (4.7)

$$\text{variance} = \rho N (2^{t/\tau})^2.$$

Therefore, the standard deviation of the population at time t becomes

$$\sigma = \sqrt{\rho N} 2^{t/\tau},$$

so that the ratio of the standard deviation to the mean becomes

$$\frac{\sigma}{\mu} = \frac{\sqrt{\rho N} 2^{t/\tau}}{\rho N 2^{t/\tau}} = \frac{1}{\sqrt{\rho N}}.$$

This is the same value for (σ/μ) that was found for the time immediate post-treatment: the relative variation in the number of resistant cells is unaffected by subsequent exponential growth. Subsequent growth to large numbers, after initial creation of a few resistant cells, will not reduce the variability between replicate experiments. Large numbers do not, per se, guarantee low relative variability. To illustrate these results we will consider a theoretical example.

Example 4.1

Consider a cell population in which drug-resistant and drug-sensitive cells grow at the same rate. Assume that drug resistance arises as a result of directed mutations and that a probe exists which can measure the number of resistant cells without affecting the system.

Consider one series of experiments in this population where the parent sensitive cells are exposed to drug at size N_1, and then the resulting resistant cells are allowed to grow for interval t. At the end, the mean and the standard deviation of the number of resistant cells is given by Equation 4.7 with $N = N_1$:

$$\mu = (\rho N_1)2^{t/\tau}$$

and

$$\sigma \sqrt{\rho N_1} 2^{t/\tau}$$

so that

$$\frac{\sigma}{\mu} = \frac{1}{\sqrt{\rho N_2}}. \tag{4.8}$$

In a second series of experiments, no drug is given at size N_1, but the parent population is permitted to grow for an interval t so that there are $N_1 2^{t/\tau}$ cells. The drug is then applied and the mean and standard deviation of the number of resistant cells produced is Equation 4.5 with $N = N_1 2^{t/\tau}$:

$$\mu = \rho(N_1 2^{t/\tau})$$

and

$$\sigma = \sqrt{\rho N_1 2^{t/\tau}},$$

so that

$$\frac{\sigma}{\mu} = \sqrt{\frac{\rho}{N_1 2^{t/\tau}}}. \tag{4.9}$$

Comparing these two series of equations we see that giving the drug earlier (Equation 4.8) versus giving it later (Equation 4.9) does not affect the mean number of resistant cells and the mean is the same for any time of administration prior to evaluation. Conversely the standard deviation is influenced by the time of administration and increases for earlier times ($\sqrt{\rho N_1} 2^{t/\tau} > \sqrt{\rho N_1 2^{t/\tau}}$). This effect is maximized when the drug is given when the parent population is sufficiently small that there are usually no resistant cells produced except rarely, when a single cell is produced which subsequently grows to form a very large population at the time of evaluation.

Random mutation model

Having developed some basic relationships for the behaviour of the directed mutation model we now wish to undertake a similar analysis of the random mutation model. Analogously to our consideration of the directed mutation model we would assume that at any time drug-sensitive cells have a common rate of acquiring resistance. It is necessary to be rather delicate in the way in which we interpret the preceding statement. For the directed mutation model, resistance develops only at times when the cells are exposed to the drug. Therefore, the probability that a cell develops resistance, at the time of drug application, and the probability that a cell is resistant soon after application of the drug, are the same. The rate at which drug resistance occurs under the directed mutation model, ρ, is defined in terms of the number of cells present when the drug is applied. There is no single point like this for the random mutation model. However, the random mutation model must behave, conceptually, like a directed mutation model in which drug is continuously applied but no sensitive cells are killed. If we use the symbol α to represent the 'rate' at which cells are 'converted' to drug resistance in the random mutational model (to distinguish it from the rate under the directed model), then we can use a differential form of the directed mutation model Equation 4.3 as a prototype for the random mutation model. We can write

$$\frac{dR}{dN} = \alpha, \qquad (4.10)$$

where dN now represents an increase in the number of sensitive cells rather than the number exposed to the drug.

It is implicit from Equation 4.10 that population growth is necessary before resistance can occur. This is not the only way to formulate the random mutational model. An alternative approach to defining the equations governing the acquisition of resistance in the random mutation model is to consider the rate α as a time-specific rate, which may be written as

$$\frac{dR}{dt} = \alpha N, \qquad (4.11)$$

where R and N (the number of sensitive cells) are dependent upon t. This particular formulation has been used extensively in other applications where it is necessary to model random creation and growth (e.g.

cosmic rays entering the earth's atmosphere). For exponentially growing cell populations, the two formulations are essentially equivalent since the rate of growth of the parent population is proportional to its size. Where the growth of the parent population is not exponential this is no longer true; however, for the purposes of this chapter we will consider the two formulations as equivalent, and will use them interchangeably. If sensitive cells did not replicate, N would not change over time and Equation 4.10 would predict that no new resistant cells would be created. However, if resistance acquisition is time dependent (Equation 4.11) then more resistant cells would be continuously produced despite the lack of growth of the sensitive cells (see also Chapter 5).

The mathematical formulation of the random selection model contained in Equation 4.11 is incomplete in two ways: (a) it only models the conversion of sensitive cells to resistance and does not include the intrinsic growth of the resistant cells and (b) it is still only formulated as a deterministic model and not a probabilistic model. The first concern is easy to address and comes by adding a term representing the intrinsic growth of already existing resistant cells, as follows

$$\frac{dR}{dt} = \alpha N + \lambda R, \tag{4.12}$$

where λ represents the intrinsic growth rate of the resistant cells ($\lambda = \ln(2)/\tau$ where τ is the doubling time). Placing this model into a rigorous probabilistic framework is complex, and we will return to this below. However, it turns out that the formulation developed to this point can be used to distinguish between the random and the directed models, as will be seen below.

Earlier we postulated that the random mutation model should behave like a directed mutation model where we continuously apply drug to the parent population and cause conversion to resistance but do not cause death of sensitive cells. We found, in our discussion of the directed mutation model, that the mean number of resistant cells present at a particular point did not depend on the (earlier) time of application of the drug but that the standard deviation did. In particular, we found that the standard deviation increased if the drug was applied earlier. Combining these observations we would deduce that the standard deviation of the number of resistant cells under the random mutation model will be greater than that under the directed mutation model in the case where they both predict the same mean number.

To illustrate this, imagine that we separate the growth of the cell population into a series of nonoverlapping adjoining time intervals of equal length Δt. Any resistant cell present at the end can trace its origin back to a progenitor resistant cell that first arose in one of these intervals. If growth is well synchronized cells will divide at the same time and it is convenient to choose the intervals to represent a single doubling (Fig. 4.2). In each interval the development of resistant cells can be expected to behave as a directed mutation process with parameter α so that (see Equation 4.4) the number of resistant cells created from previously sensitive cells using a Poisson distribution with a mean, μ, is given by

$$\mu = \alpha \Delta N, \tag{4.13}$$

where ΔN is the increase in cell number associated with the doubling in the interval. The increase in cell number ΔN is given by

$$\Delta N = N_0 e^{\lambda(t+\Delta t)} - N_0 e^{\lambda t} = N_0 e^{\lambda t}(e^{\lambda \Delta t} - 1), \tag{4.14}$$

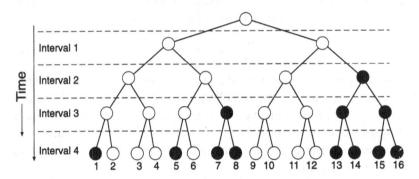

Fig. 4.2. The growth of a hypothetical cell population originating from a single cell is depicted through four consecutive synchronous divisions causing it to increase to 16 cells. The history of the cell division and growth is divided into four time intervals separating different generational divisions. Resistant cells (indicated by solid circles) are assumed to arise via random mutations that occur with certain probability at each division of a sensitive cell. Of the 16 cells present after four divisions, eight are resistant. For each of the resistant cells (cells numbered 1, 5, 7, 8, 13, 14, 15, 16) it is possible to trace back its lineage until the progenitor resistant cell is identified. Each progenitor cell will have arisen in one of the disjoint intervals defined by the divisions of each of the cells. Thus resistant cells 1 and 5 have first resistant progenitors in interval 4 (themselves); 7 and 8 have a common resistant progenitor in interval 3 and 13, 14, 15 and 16 have a common resistant progenitor in interval 2.

that is the difference in the number of cells at the beginning ($N_0 e^{\lambda t}$) and the number of cells at the end ($N_0 e^{\lambda(t+\Delta t)}$) of the interval. Combining Equations 4.13 and 4.14, the mean number of resistant cells that arise from pre-existing sensitive cells in this interval is

$$\mu = \alpha \times N_0 e^{\lambda t}(e^{\lambda \Delta t} - 1). \tag{4.15}$$

Now we may use Equation 4.15 to calculate the expected number of resistant cells, μ^*, present at a later time t^*, which are derived from new resistant cells created in this interval. This is obtained by multiplying Equation 4.15 by the mean increase in growth over the subsequent interval of length ($t^* - t - \Delta t$), which is $e^{\lambda(t^*-t-\Delta t)}$, so that

$$\mu^* = \alpha N_0 e^{\lambda t}(e^{\lambda \Delta t} - 1) \times e^{\lambda(t^*-t-\Delta t)} = \alpha N_0 e^{\lambda t^*}(1 - e^{-\lambda \Delta t}). \tag{4.16}$$

But it can be seen from Equation 4.16 that μ^* depends only on the length of the interval, Δt, and the final time t^* and not the time of the beginning of the interval, t, since t does not appear in the equation. Hence the formula applies to any of the intervals, showing that two intervals, of the same length, make an identical 'contribution' to the overall mean number of resistant cells. However, earlier intervals have greater variability in the number of cells they contribute at time t^* as we will now show.

Using the same approach as before, in which we cut the history of the tumour into a series of disjoint time intervals, we can calculate the overall variance. Since resistance occurring in one cell in an earlier interval implies that its progeny in a later interval are already resistant, each interval is not statistically independent of another. However, this dependence is slight and we will assume that the resistance arising in each interval is independent of others. Under the assumption of independence, the overall variance at time t^* is just the sum of the variances that each preceding interval contributes. Let $(\sigma^*)^2$ be the contribution to the variance at time t^* for one interval of length Δt commencing at time t (μ^* was the contribution to the mean). If the interval length is sufficiently short, then the number of resistant cells in the interval is just equal to the number that have spontaneously converted from sensitivity, since they will have had no time for further growth. The variance of the number of new resistant cells converting in an interval is given by the variance of the Poisson distribution, which is equal to its mean and is given in Equation 4.15. In order to calculate its contribution to the overall variance at time t^*, we multiply this by the square of the mean regrowth subsequent to the interval: $[e^{\lambda((t^*-t-\Delta t)}]^2$ (see Equation 4.7). Accordingly

$$
\begin{aligned}
(\sigma^*)^2 &= \alpha N_0 e^{\lambda t}(e^{\lambda \Delta t} - 1) \times [e^{\lambda(t^*-t-\Delta t)}]^2 \\
&= \alpha N_0 e^{\lambda t}(e^{\lambda \Delta t} - 1) \times e^{2\lambda(t^*-t-\Delta t)} \\
&= \alpha N_0 (1 - e^{-\lambda \Delta t})e^{\lambda t^*} \times e^{\lambda(t^*-t-\Delta t)} \\
&= \mu^* \times e^{\lambda(t^*-t-\Delta t)}.
\end{aligned}
$$

We can see that the above formula multiplies the contribution to the mean, μ^*, by a factor that increases for intervals earlier in the period (smaller t). When we sum over the $(\sigma^*)^2$ terms for each interval to form the total variance we find that it is greater than the overall mean because of multiplication by these factors, $e^{\lambda(t^*-t-\Delta t)}$. We obtain the result that under the random mutation model the variance of the number of resistant cells exceeds its mean at the time of drug application.

Implications of the analysis

The directed mutation model predicts that, immediately after drug application, the number of resistant cells follows a Poisson distribution with the variance equal to the mean, μ; whereas the random mutation model predicts that the distribution of resistant cells has a variance that is greater than the mean μ.

This is an extremely important point. It is a mathematical property of the Poisson distribution that its mean is equal to its variance. In the case of a *directed mutation* process there is a single event (and hence a single Poisson distribution) that results in the generation of resistant cells. In a *random* mutational process there are a series of what we might call mini-Poisson events, each with its own mean and variance. These random events are then propagated by the growth of the resistant cells and continue to occur until the drug is applied and the selection of the resistant cells occurs.

Having identified this distinction between the two models, Luria and Delbrück proceeded to develop an experimental method in which the results are sensitive to the relationship between the mean and the variance. They called their method the *fluctuation test*.

4.5   The fluctuation test

Since its introduction in 1943, the fluctuation test has been modified in a number of ways to suit individual experimental conditions. Its essential nature is unchanged and will be outlined here. A schematic description is given in Fig. 4.3. First a parental line of wild-type cells is obtained and divided into two equal samples A and B. Sample B is then divided to provide a large number, n say, of equally sized portions, or aliquots. The size of the aliquot is selected so that the likelihood of resistant cells being present is small and, where possible, the size is sufficient for regular growth to be expected. Sample A and Sample B are then grown under identical conditions until they have reached a size where approximately one resistant cell can be expected to be present in each aliquot of sample B (if the random mutation hypothesis is true) or one resistant cell would be induced by application of the drug if the directed mutation model is true. At this point, sample A is mixed to minimize any inhomogeneities and divided into n aliquots, so that Sample A and Sample B both consist of n equal sized portions. If the growth process is not perfectly regular then the initial aliquots in sample B may vary in size substantially at the time of drug exposure. If this is the case then Sample A should be divided to have the same distribution of sizes as Sample B. Throughout this process each sample has been maintained in as identical a condition as possible. For simplicity we will refer to the portions drawn from each sample as Sample A and Sample B. Drug is now added to each of the samples to produce resistance (directed model) or select for resistance (random model). Drug-sensitive cells are eliminated and only the resistant ones remain. At this point each sample is homogenized and plated individually onto an appropriate medium. Cells are allowed to grow and the number of clones formed is counted. Each clone is assumed to originate from a single drug-resistant cell and the number of clones grown from each sample equals the number of drug-resistant cells present after exposure to the drug. The mean number of drug-resistant cells in the aliquots of Sample A and Sample B are calculated and the variance between aliquots within each sample computed.

The two samples experience identical experimental conditions except that Sample A is divided after growth and shortly prior to drug administration whereas Sample B is grown after division into aliquots. How does this provide a method for distinguishing between the induction and selection models? The approach taken by Luria and Delbrück in

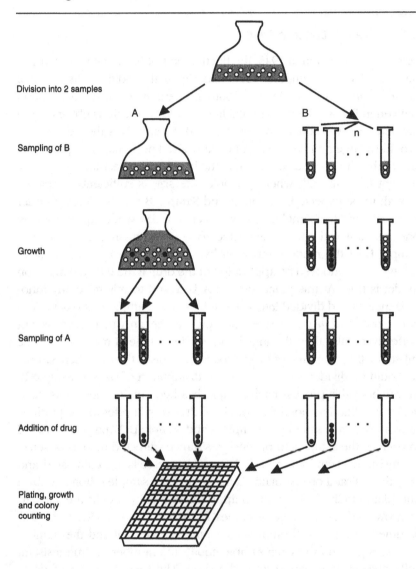

Fig. 4.3. The overall pattern of the fluctuation test is depicted in this figure. First two equal sized populations are drawn from a homogenized parent population. One is placed in a single flask (Sample A) whilst the second is divided into n subsamples (Sample B). Both samples are then allowed to grow in identical conditions until the average size of the population in each subsample in B reaches a critical size (where there would be approximately one resistant cell present). At this point, Sample A is mixed and then divided into n separate subsamples, which should be of the same average size as those in Sample B. Each subsample (in both A and B) is then exposed to the

their fluctuation test was to demonstrate that the standard deviation was inflated by a selection mechanism in Sample B by incorporating an internal control which would provide a separate estimate of the variance under a Poisson model. This control was provided by the portions from Sample A. The cells in Sample A aliquots were exposed to the same conditions as those from B except that they were divided into portions immediately prior to drug exposure. Consider the effect of this process under the two models.

Under the directed mutation model, prior to drug exposure, each aliquot (whether from Sample A or Sample B) consists of a uniform sample of sensitive cells. After drug is applied, each contains a random number of resistant cells. The distribution of that number of resistant cells is given by Equation 4.4 and has a mean and standard deviation given by Equation 4.5. This distribution is the same for aliquots from both samples and only depends upon the size of the aliquot at drug exposure, N.

Under the random mutation model prior to division, Sample A consists of an inhomogeneous mixture of sensitive and resistant cells. Homogenizing and division into aliquots results in each aliquot having a random number of resistant cells. The expected (mean) number of resistant cells in each aliquot is the same (call it μ') and is equal to the total number of resistant cells (R_A) in Sample A divided by the number of aliquots, n, that is $\mu' = R_A/n$. The process of mixing and random sampling implies that the resulting distribution will have a Poisson form with parameter R_A/n. The variance of the number of resistant cells per aliquot from Sample A is thus also R_A/n (since it has a Poisson distribution). The variance between aliquots in Sample A is equal (on average) to the within aliquot variance, so that the variance in the number of surviving resistant cells after drug administration will be R_A/n for Sample A.

Caption for Fig. 4.3 (*cont.*)
drug. Sensitive cells are killed and only resistant cells survive. Surviving resistant cells are counted, either by plating or by some other method. The count of the number of surviving resistant cells per subsample is noted and the variation in counts for each sample calculated. Under the directed mutation model, similar variation in counts is expected in each sample whereas the variation for Sample B is expected to exceed that for Sample A under the random mutation model.

Sample B represents n independent aliquots, each of which has developed a random number of resistant cells. Defining R_B to represent the sum of the numbers of resistant cells in all the n aliquots from Sample B, then each aliquot has the same expected number of resistant cells, R_B/n. However, as described on p. 105, each aliquot from sample B has a variance that exceeds its mean, R_B/n. Since the two samples contain the same numbers of cells and all conditions have been kept as similar as possible, the two samples should contain the same average aggregate number of resistant cells, i.e. the mean of R_A is the same as the mean of R_B. Finally, we deduce that under the random mutation model the variance between the aliquots (which is, on average, the same as the variance of each aliquot) is greater for Sample B than for Sample A, whereas they are the same under the directed mutation model.

In summary, under the directed mutation model the aliquots from Samples A and B both have the same (Poisson) distribution of resistant cells. Under the random mutation model, the aliquots from Sample A and Sample B have different distributions of resistant cells; in particular the variance in Sample B exceeds that of Sample A.

4.6   Analysis of data from the fluctuation test

The beauty of the fluctuation test is that it reduces a complex problem to a simple test. The statistical procedure used to analyse data from these experiments is known as ANOVA (**analysis of variance**). This test compares groups of means from various samples to determine whether some means are more widely separated than others. In this case, the means are the individual aliquot counts and we wish to determine whether the counts in aliquots from Sample A are less widely separated than the counts from sample B. This technique is widely used in statistics and a large number of statistical software packages exist that contain it. This method does not rely on the Poisson distribution but only compares the variance between aliquots of the two samples.

4.7   Experiment of Lederberg and Lederberg

In 1952 Joshua and Ethel Lederberg described an ingenious method for evaluating whether resistance arose through random or directed adaptation. Their experiment was basically to utilize a bacterial culture plate that was covered with colonies of *Escherichia coli* and then employ a sterilized tube covered with velvet nap, which was brought into contact with the plate. Some of the cells adhered to the nap and when this was brought into contact with a second plate a portion of cells were transferred in such a way as to preserve their original spacing and spatial orientation. The second culture plate could then be treated with bacteria-lysing phage or with antibiotics.

As cells are not mobile on the culture plate, adjacent cells are much more likely to share common ancestors than cells distant from one another. If that common ancestor was resistant then cells at the same location on each plate will be resistant. If the total population has not been previously exposed to the drug then the directed mutation model would imply that there were no pre-existing resistant cells. If the two plates are now exposed to drug then this model would imply that there would be no systematic correlation between the spatial patterns of surviving cells on the two plates other than that which could be attributed to chance. The random mutation model implies that pre-existing resistant cells will be present prior to transference so that there will exist some correlation in the patterns of surviving clones on the two plates.

It will be remembered that in the fluctuation test any possibility of spatial relationships among evolving populations of bacteria will be disrupted by both the circumstances of growing the bacteria in a liquid medium and the process of careful mixing. Conceptually, the Lederbergs' 'blue velvet' experiment is probably easier to understand than the fluctuation test and it is an elegant method for demonstrating the prior existence of mutant forms.

Lederberg and Lederberg presented no mathematical analysis so that it would be possible to analyse the data from such an experiment to distinguish between directed and random mutation models. Despite the method's conceptual simplicity, the analysis is complicated by the sampling variation present in cell transference between the plates. However it is straightforward to see how a variation of this method could be analysed using currently available technology. Instead of using a plate, the cells are individually transferred to microwells, with one cell in each. The cells then double once and one cell from each well is transferred to a second plate of microwells, with each cell going to the same well position on the new plate that it occupied previously. Each microwell on both plates is then exposed to the same level of drug and the locations of surviving clones on each plate is recorded (Fig. 4.4). Let there be M microwells on each plate and let r_1 and r_2 resistant cells be observed

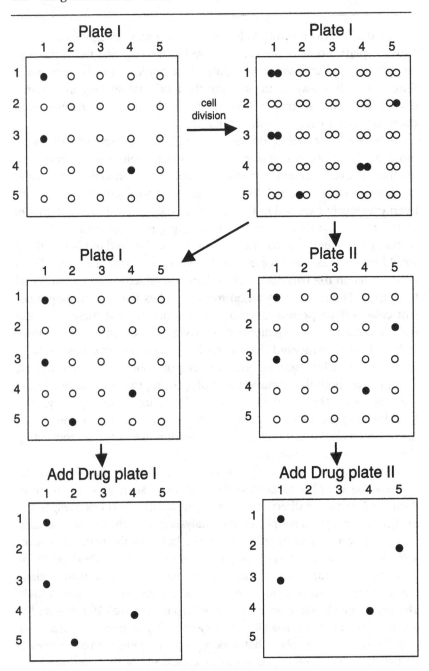

on plates 1 and 2, respectively. Under the directed mutation model, the distribution of resistant cells on each plate will be random and the likelihood that the same well location on both plates will have a resistant cell is

$$\frac{r_1}{M} \times \frac{r_2}{M}.$$

Therefore, there will, on average, be

$$M \times \frac{r_1}{M} \times \frac{r_2}{M} \tag{4.17}$$

wells that have resistant cells at the same location on both plates under the directed mutation model. The number of wells that have resistant cells on both plates is approximately Poisson distributed so that the variance of this random variable is also given by Equation 4.17.

Under the random mutation model, prior to division there will be r', say, pre-existing resistant cells, which each divide to form resistant cells in the same location on each plate. In addition, there will be more resistant cells created at division, $\Delta r'$, which will be randomly divided between the two plates. Now by definition each of the sites where one of the r' pre-existing resistant cells existed will have a resistant cell at the same location on the other plate and none of the $\Delta r'$ sites, where

Fig. 4.4. In this idealized version of the Lederberg and Lederberg (1952) experiment, an array of cells is created by placing individual cells in wells. Each microwell contains the same number of cells (one cell in the illustration). The location of each cell can be identified by the coordinates of the well. In the illustration, the centre well has location (3,3). Each cell is allowed to double so that there are now two cells in each well. One cell from each well is then drawn at random and placed in the same coordinate location that it previously occupied on a second plate, thus creating two identical plates each with one cell per microwell in the same location. These cells are then exposed to drug and the surviving cells (open circles) are identified and their coordinates noted. Under the directed mutation model there will be few surviving cells (resistant) at the same coordinates on each plate. Under the random mutation model the possibility that resistance may have been pre-existing increases the probability that there will be resistant cells at the same locations.

resistant cells were created, will have resistant cells at the same well on both plates. Thus there will be r' wells that have resistant cells on both plates under the random mutation model, in contrast to that predicted for the directed mutation model in Equation 4.17. Since the total number of resistant cells on both plates must equal the observed number, we must have,

$$r_1 + r_2 = 2r' + \Delta r, \qquad (4.18)$$

with both r_1 and r_2 greater than r'. We expect the number of wells containing resistant cells on both plates to be much greater under the random mutation model than under the directed mutation model, i.e.

$$r' > M \times \frac{r_1}{M} \times \frac{r_2}{M},$$

as the following example illustrates.

Example 4.2

Consider a case where there are 10 000 wells and 1 in 1000 wells contains a resistant cell. Then under the directed model we would expect

$$M \times \frac{r_1}{M} \times \frac{r_2}{M} = 10\,000 \times \frac{1}{1000} \times \frac{1}{1000} = 0.01$$

wells per experiment to contain resistant cells on both plates. Therefore, only about 1 in 100 such experiments would have resistant cells at the same site on both plates. Under the random mutation model there will be r' such wells; but what magnitude is r' expected to be? Now since equal intervals contribute equal numbers of resistant cells (Equation 4.16 and preceding discussion) we know that $2r' > \Delta r$. Substituting this inequality into Equation 4.18 gives

$$r_1 + r_2 < 2r' + 2r,$$

so that we have $r' > (r_1 + r_2)/4$. Now with 10 000 wells and 1 in 1000 resistant cells, each plate will have approximately 10 resistant cells; we would expect r' to exceed 5((10 + 10)/4). Therefore, under the random mutation model one would expect to find wells on both plates with resistant cells while under the directed model this would be rare.

Although this technique provides a quite powerful way to distinguish between the random and the directed mutational models, it can be seen that the magnitude of the experiments involved may make them impractical. Spatial inhomogeneity in the distribution of resistant cells is one of the principal predictions of a random mutation model.

4.8   Applications of the fluctuation test to cancer chemotherapy

The preceding discussion may be termed 'classical' in that it represents the use of the tests in determining resistance in bacterial populations to either drugs or viral infection. Its application to *in vitro* tumour systems is little different in that such cells may be manipulated in ways similar to that of bacterial populations. Therefore, many examples of the fluctuation test are available from the literature for *in vitro* tumour systems. The results of such experiments almost all support a random mutation model for the origin of drug-resistant mutants in *in vitro* tumour systems. Although such observations do not prove that resistant phenotypes arise only via random mutation, such cells do seem to be the predominant type. In many cases where the creation of resistant cells does not seem to be via random mutations, selection takes place at high drug doses and the cells do not maintain their resistance. This suggests such resistance is related to some epigenetic phenomenon that permits the stochastic survival of a few cells. It must be emphasized that a positive fluctuation test does not exclude the existence of directed mutations but it does indicate that random mutations are more common.

Clearly the experimental nature of the fluctuation test makes it impossible to use it to determine the origins of cellular resistance to chemotherapy in clinical cancer. However, its application to experimental tumour systems in animals is possible. The complexity and cost of such an undertaking has resulted in comparatively few studies being made. One published study has reported results compatible with a random mutation hypothesis (Law, 1952), while a second unpublished one has reported equivocal results (H. Lloyd and H.E. Skipper, unpublished, 1972). The design of these two studies is similar but they contained one major modification of the fluctuation test used by Luria and Delbrück (1943).

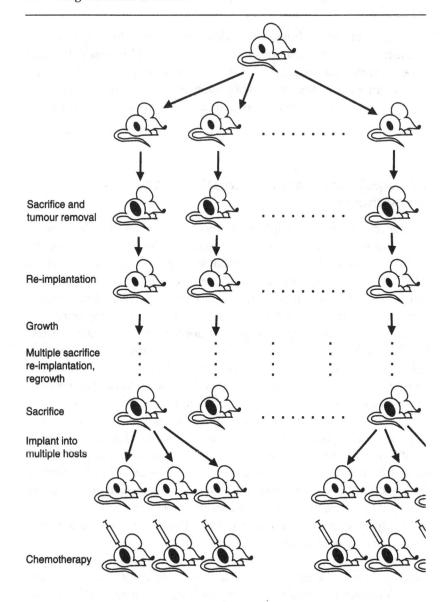

Sacrifice and
tumour removal

Re-implantation

Growth

Multiple sacrifice
re-implantation,
regrowth

Sacrifice

Implant into
multiple hosts

Chemotherapy

Observe outcome

Fig. 4.5 An initial parent tumour is removed from a host, homogenized and
re-implanted, at a smaller inoculum size, into a number of new hosts. The
tumour is then allowed to grow until it reaches a critical size (usually
determined by the growth curve of the tumour and the capacity of the animal
to carry the tumour) when it is harvested, homogenized and a subsample

4.9   In vivo fluctuation tests

The first study was reported by Law in 1952, while H. Lloyd and H.E. Skipper carried out a similar study (personal communication) in 1972.

In both studies the L1210 leukaemia line was used in DBA mice. The experiment by Law examined resistance to amethopterin (methotrexate) and the experiments performed by Lloyd and Skipper analysed resistance to O-palmityl ara-C. In each case multiple sublines were cultured from a single line and repeatedly passaged through animal hosts (seven times in Law's experiments and 11 times in Skipper and Lloyd's) separately maintaining each subline. Passaging involved implanting a constant sized inoculum and allowing this to grow to a fixed size, sacrificing the host, harvesting the tumour and extracting a new inoculum for re-implantation to a new host. After this had been done the number of times required by the experiment, multiple inocula from the tumour were created and implanted separately into animals. The host animals were then treated with the prescribed chemotherapy and the results noted. The structure of these experiments is given schematically in Fig. 4.5. In the experiments by Law, tumour weight was the primary outcome, based on sacrifice data obtained at a fixed time postchemotherapy. Skipper and Lloyd's experiments utilized median survival time and surviving fraction as outcomes. In both series of experiments one subline was considered to be a control.

In terms of our previous description of the fluctuation test, the control subline represented sample A whereas the remaining test sublines represent sample B. In order that the final measurements be carried out on similar numbers of animals in A and B, the control subline had a larger

Caption to Fig. 4.5 (*cont.*)
re-implanted in a single new host. This cycle of growth, harvesting and implantation is then repeated several times. At the completion of this the tumour is harvested and each subline is re-implanted into an equal number of animals except for the 'control' subline where the tumour is implanted into a larger number of animals. Subsequent to re-implantation, the tumour is allowed to grow a common time and then each animal receives chemotherapy. Depending on the study design, various endpoints are measured: survival of the animal, time to death, tumour weight at some fixed later time. These endpoints are then compared between the control subline and other sublines.

number of inocula prepared from it for implanting into the animals receiving chemotherapy than the test sublines. In all cases the inoculum size was the same. The above description, not considering quantitative specifications of doses, inoculum sizes, etc., summarizes the plan of these studies. Other ancillary studies were conducted to verify that the original tumour line did not contain 'too many' resistant cells and that the sublines maintained their malignant potential after passaging.

Before considering the differences between these two experiments, first consider the difference between them and the 'classic fluctuation test'. The most obvious difference is the serial transplantation of (each) sublines through the hosts. This is required by the host-dependent nature of tumour growth, but why was repeat serial transplantation done? Neither of the reports explains why such repeat passaging was done. The report by Law was published first and, since this did provide unambiguous indication for the random mutation model for methotrexate resistance in L1210, the same design may have just been replicated by Skipper and Lloyd. The main mechanism by which the random mutation model leads to a greater variance than the directed model is the influence of the early transformations to resistance. An early transformation may be defined in terms of the probability of no transformations having occurred. This probability declines from unity to zero as the tumour grows. If, at the stage of growth of the tumour, this probability exceeds 0.95 then an existing resistant cell may be termed an 'early' transformation. Similarly if the first transformation occurs after the probability has declined below 0.05 it may be termed late. As has already been shown, early events disproportionately influence the variance.

Repeat passaging will influence the effect of early transformations under the random mutation model in two potential ways. Firstly, if the inoculum size for re-implantation is too small then it will not contain any resistant cells and only sensitive cells will be implanted. Secondly, if the inocula size is too large then it will always contain resistant cells so that a resistant tumour will always be re-implanted. Therefore, unless the inocula are in the correct size range, the procedure of serial passaging in this way will tend to produce a homogeneous result. It seems more likely to err on the side of drawing too small samples than too large samples because one requires some variability at final analysis and it is always possible to obtain resistance in a sensitive subline but not the converse. Serial passaging outside the optimum range of sizes may actually tend to remove the effect of the all-important early transformations or provide too much opportunity for them to occur. Both influences will tend to diminish differences between the sublines. From this analysis, it is certainly clear that the effect of serial passaging will depend on the inoculum size, tumour size at animal sacrifice and the value of α.

A further factor to consider in understanding these experiments is the different measures of outcome that were used. Law measured tumour weight in animals at a fixed time postchemotherapy. Skipper and Lloyd measured median survival time and surviving proportion. We would expect tumour weight to be a sensitive measure to use in the fluctuation test since it is directly proportional to the number of cells present, which will be directly proportional to the number of resistant cells present at the completion of chemotherapy. For this reason, if there were a 100-fold range in the number of resistant cells after chemotherapy, there would be an approximate 100-fold range in tumour weights at a fixed time later. Since animals die from this tumour at about the same body burden, the time to death will also be related to the number of resistant cells after chemotherapy. However the relationship between the number of resistant cells and tumour weight is stronger than that with survival time. Similarly, the variation in survival rates may also be small, since a tumour will prove fatal ultimately if it contains 1 or 100 resistant cells.

A further difference between the 'classical' fluctuation test and the two animal experiments is the control sample. In the animal experiments a single subline was selected as the control. This differs from the classical test in that although sample A consisted of a single sample it was equal in size to the aliquots that constituted sample B. Therefore, the two samples should have the same underlying distribution of total number of resistant cells. In the animal experiments the overall proportion of resistant cells is expected to be the same in each sample but because one sample is composed of multiple sublines and the other of a single subline, the overall combined proportion will be more variable in the single subline sample than in the combined.

It would seem that these published experiments designed to mimic the fluctuation test *in vivo* possess various problems that will limit their capacity to distinguish efficiently between the two models. The fact that one of these experiments, that by Law, did show evidence of a random mutation effect must be counted as strong evidence for the existence of this as a mechanism for the production of resistance *in vivo*.

4.10   Summary and conclusions

Two models, selection and directed mutation, have been proposed for the origin of resistant cells. The selection model predicts that resistant cells are spontaneously created in the absence of a drug while the directed mutation model indicates that it is the interaction between drug and cell which creates resistant cells. In the absence of specific markers of resistance that may be accurately measured in mixed populations of cells, it is not possible to distinguish directly between these two hypotheses. An indirect method, known as the fluctuation test, makes such a separation possible. This experimental approach relies on the deduction that the selection model predicts, under uniform conditions, much greater variability in the observed number of resistant cells than the induction model does. This test has been used to show that resistance is acquired by a selection process to a large variety of drugs in *in vitro* tumour systems. Evidence from *in vivo* tumour systems is very limited but appears to be compatible with the same mechanism.

In his autobiography Salvador Luria (1983) recounted how he got the idea for the fluctuation analysis experiment. He had observed someone playing a slot machine, noticing that the player frequently got no return, occasionally a small amount and then, rarely, would 'hit the jackpot' with a large pay out. The average earnings from the machine would be quite low, but every so often by chance there would be a large sum discharged from the machine. Luria realized that the average payoff in the game would not tell the whole story, but the gambler would be interested in the rare big win that would occur. A random process like mutations would, likewise, occasionally produce a 'jackpot' owing to the mutant arising very early in the expansion of a clonal population. Intuitively recognizing that this would be the case was one thing, but rigorously proving it scientifically was something else. At that juncture, Luria called upon his colleague Max Delbrück, a physicist, to help with the statistical analysis of the data that would allow a distinction to be made between an induced or a spontaneous event.

The fluctuation test is one of the most ingenious biological experiments ever devised. The assumptions that go into it are very subtle and a full mathematical discussion of the theory would go well beyond the algebra and basic calculus used in this chapter.

We can say that whatever other processes may be operative to produce drug resistance, clearly spontaneous mutations are one of them.

Although a number of the therapeutic implications are the same for both an induction and a mutation model, there are important areas of difference. A 'naive' induction model would argue that the tumour cells exist in some kind of indeterminate state with respect to drug-resistance markers prior to drug exposure. Looking for them prior to treatment would be pointless (presumably no one would suggest that the act of histological staining can induce these markers in dead cells). However, if prior information about the resistance profile of the tumour can be obtained without *in vivo* destructive testing then clearly this will be important.

References

Burnett, F.M. (1929). 'Smooth–rough' variation in bacteria and its relation to bacteriophage. *J. Path. Bact.*, 32: 15–42.

Law, L.W. (1952). Origin of the resistance of leukemic cells to folic acid antagonists. *Nature*, 169: 628–629.

Lederberg, J. and Lederberg, E.M. (1952). Replica plating and indirect selection of bacterial mutants. *J. Bacteriol.*, 3: 399–406.

Luria, S.E. (1983). *A Slot Machine, a Broken Test Tube.* Harper & Rowe, New York.

Luria, S.E. and Delbrück, M. (1943). Mutations of bacteria from virus sensitivity to virus resistance. *Genetics*, 28: 491–511.

Further reading

Armitage, P. (1952). The statistical theory of bacterial populations subject to mutation. *J. R. Stat. Soc.(B)*, 14: 1–33.

Lea, D.E. and Coulson, C.A. (1948). The distribution of the number of mutants in bacterial populations. *J. Genetics*, 49: 264–285.

Ling, V. (1982). Genetic basis of drug resistance in mammalian cells. In *Drug and Hormone Resistance in Neoplasia*, Vol. 1, *Basic Concepts*, ed. N. Bruchovsky and J.H. Goldie, pp. 1–19. CRC Press, Boca Raton, FL.

Luria, S.E. (1951). The frequency distribution of sponanteous bacteriophage mutants as evidence for the exponential rate of phage reproduction. *Cold Spring Harbor Symp. Quant. Biol.*, 16: 463–470.

Snedecor, G.W. and Cochrane, W.G. (1967). *Statistical Methods*, 6th edn, Ch. 10. Iowa State Press, Ames, IA.

5

Development and exploration of the random mutation model for drug resistance

5.1 Introduction

In this chapter, we further develop the description of resistance in quantitative terms. Chapter 4 detailed how the quantitative analysis of the directed and random mutation models for the development of drug resistance provided a method, the fluctuation test, to distinguish between them. Evidence was cited that favoured the random mutation model, implying that the onset of resistance would be a variable process and would occur prior to application of the drug. However, it is worth noting that many of the deductions that we will make will be equally true under a directed mutation model.

In the development that follows, we will assume that resistance arises via a random mutation process. The purpose of this chapter is to develop equations which describe the evolution of the resistant cell compartment as the tumour grows when resistance is caused by random mutations.

In order to discuss resistance in tumour systems one must first have some basic model for the functioning of the tumour system. A basic model for functioning will mean widely different things to different people, but here we will be concerned about the way in which the tumour system grows. We will be concentrating on a quantitative description of the growth of resistant and sensitive cell populations without detailed description of what regulates or stimulates such growth. We believe this approach is justified in that it permits concentration on the dynamics of the resistance process; however, as with any other model, such simplification is justified only if it does not lead to erroneous conclusions. We use the term *model* to imply some construct intended to describe reality. The models we will discuss are mainly conceptual and mathematical although we will frequently make reference to physical models.

5.2   Exponential model of tumour growth and the expected number of resistant cells

Consider first the overall growth of the malignant cell population without worrying whether such cells are sensitive or resistant. Cell growth proceeds by a process of binary fission. The time from creation of a cell to the time it divides to form two new cells is called the *division time*. If the division time is perfectly stable and cells continue dividing then the resultant growth is known mathematically as *geometric*. Fortunately, cell growth in real populations is not totally synchronous so that after a few divisions cells are sufficiently out of step that the population is increasing steadily rather than in large jumps. In this case, it becomes reasonable to think of the growth process as proceeding smoothly and regularly over time. Not only does this make for good looking graphs but it permits much easier mathematical analysis. Smoothly changing functions may be analysed using calculus; the methods for analysing processes which change by variable integer increments are not nearly so elegant. The smooth equivalent of geometric growth is *exponential growth* (see also Chapter 2). The mathematical description of exponential growth may be written in a number of different ways, with mathematicians favouring a form like

$$N(t) = N_0 e^{\lambda t} \qquad (5.1)$$

where t represents time and N_0 is the number of cells at $t = 0$. An alternative, and in this context more suggestive, way to put this equation is

$$N(t) = 2^{t/\tau},$$

where τ is the division time of the cells (synonymous with generation time, cell cycle time, intermitotic time, the time required to move from one mitosis (M phase) to the next; see p. 45). The above equations imply that fractions of cells are present most of the time since $N(t)$ will be a whole number for few values of t. However this inconvenience is ignored because the number of cells is usually large.

A defining characteristic of exponential growth is that the rate of growth is proportional to the population size. Using calculus, the rate of growth is denoted by dN/dt and we have the usual defining equation for the exponential

$$\frac{dN}{dt} = \lambda N(t), \qquad (5.2)$$

i.e. the rate of growth of each cell is the same so that the overall rate of growth is proportional to the tumour size.

In order to continue further and incorporate the existence of resistant cells, we need to develop linked equations that describe the growth of the sensitive and resistant cells. Denote the number of sensitive cells at time t by $S(t)$ and the number of resistant cells by $R(t)$, then

$$N(t) = S(t) + R(t)$$

since each cell must be either sensitive or resistant by assumption. If resistant and sensitive cells grow and divide in the same way, the same type of equation (as Equation 5.2) will hold for both types of cell to describe their intrinsic growth, i.e. $dS/dt = \lambda S(t)$ etc. If the two types grow exponentially but at different rates, then we would use a different λ value for each cell type (or in the equivalent growth equation a different τ). An exponential growth model provides the most basic mathematical model for describing the growth of pre-existing sensitive and resistant cells.

In order to describe fully the growth of the sensitive and resistant cell compartments, we must not only describe their own intrinsic growth but also the transformation of sensitive cells to resistant cells. In Section 4.4 we considered two formulations for the random mutation model (Equations 4.10 and 4.11) in which α was viewed as either a division- or time-dependent rate. If divisions occur regularly in time then it is possible to use either formulation so that, under such circumstances, the two formulations are mathematically equivalent. However, it must be noted that they do not necessarily say the same thing. A time-dependent rate may imply that elapsed time has some direct effect on the development of resistance whereas a division-dependent rate implies that it is movement through the cell cycle which drives the development of resistance. We favour the latter model and use it throughout this book. When growth is regular it is often convenient to convert the division-specific rate into a per unit time rate since

rate of resistance per unit time =
rate of resistance per unit division × division rate

In our case we have

rate of resistance per unit time = rate of resistance per unit division × λ.

Consider now the expected growth of the resistant cells. If, as before, α is the rate of resistance acquisition per cell division and there are $S(t)$ sensitive cells present, then new resistant cells are arising via transformation at rate

$$\alpha \lambda S(t).$$

If the resistant cells have the same intrinsic growth rate as the sensitive cells then existing resistant cells are growing at rate

$$\lambda R(t).$$

The overall growth rate of the number of resistant cells, dR/dt, is given by the sum of the intrinsic growth rate plus that resulting from new transformations, i.e.

$$\frac{dR}{dt} = \lambda R(t) + \alpha \lambda S(t). \tag{5.3}$$

We cannot solve this equation for $R(t)$ since we do not know what $S(t)$ is, so we must first find it. We have exactly the same equation for the growth of the sensitive cells except we now subtract the cells, $\alpha \lambda S(t)$, that are transferring from sensitivity to resistance, i.e.

$$\frac{dS}{dt} = \lambda S(t) - \alpha \lambda S(t) = \lambda[1 - \alpha]S(t). \tag{5.4}$$

Equation 5.4 may be solved since it only includes terms in $S(t)$ and is nothing but the defining equation for an exponential, with a rate constant $\lambda[1 - \alpha]$. Since $\alpha \ll 1$ (much less than 1), the term $[1 - \alpha]$ is frequently approximated by 1 so that we have

$$\frac{dS}{dt} = \lambda S(t),$$

which has the solution:

$$S(t) = S_0 e^{\lambda t}, \tag{5.5}$$

where S_0 is the number of sensitive cells at time $t = 0$. If we now substitute the solution in Equation 5.5 into Equation 5.3 for $R(t)$ then we have

$$\frac{dR}{dt} = \lambda R(t) + \alpha \lambda S_0 e^{\lambda t},$$

which has as its solution

$$R(t) = R_0 e^{\lambda t} + \alpha \lambda t S_0 e^{\lambda t}, \tag{5.6}$$

where R_0 is the number of resistant cells present at time $t = 0$. It can be seen that the formula for the number of sensitive cells is contained in the expression for the number of resistant cells, indicating the relationship between the size of each 'compartment'. (Compartment will be used to refer to groups of cells within the tumour that are homogeneous with respect to some characteristic; thus the sensitive compartment consists of all cells that are sensitive to the drug in question.)

Figure 5.1 plots $N(t)$ as given by Equation 5.1 and $R(t)$ as given in Equation 5.6 for several values of α. A log–linear scale is used so that the exponential growth of the total population appears as a straight line. In

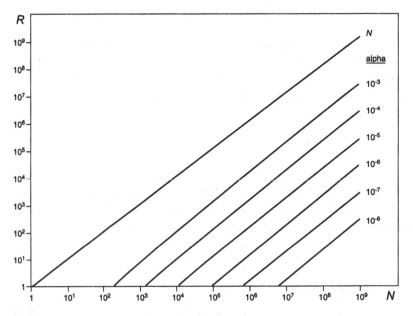

Fig. 5.1. Plot of mean number of resistant cells, R, as a function of the overall number of tumour cells, N, and the transition rate α. Both axes use logarithmic scales. The overall tumour size N is also plotted for reference. It can be seen that the values of N and α strongly influence the number of resistant cells. The proportion of resistant cells, for specific values of α, increases as the tumour grows (N increases) although this only changes slowly. As a result, it is the value of the product αN that primarily determines the expected number of resistant cells.

these illustrations, it is assumed that $N_0 = 1$ and $R_0 = 0$ so that the tumour starts from a single sensitive cell. Therefore, the resistant population starts at zero (not depicted since $\log(0) = -\infty$) and increases smoothly as time elapses (and the tumour grows). The rate of increase of the resistant population is slightly greater than that of the total population, as demonstrated by the slightly stronger gradient. If extended indefinitely the tumour would become totally resistant (for all values of α).

We now consider a short example utilizing the formulae presented.

Example 5.1

Consider an experiment in which we wish to calculate the number of resistant cells at the time of first treatment. A mouse is inoculated with 8×10^5 tumour cells from a tumour with a doubling time of 8 hours. The animal is to be exposed to a drug 72 hours later, for which the random mutation rate is $\alpha = 1 \times 10^{-7}$ per cell division. To proceed, first we calculate the value of λ. We have stated before that

$$e^{\lambda t} = 2^{t/\tau},$$

since these are two alternative formulations of the same equation. Taking logarithms to the base e on both sides of this equation gives

$$\lambda t = \frac{t}{\tau}\ln(2),$$

$$\lambda = \frac{1}{\tau}\ln(2),$$

where ln represents logarithms to the base e. Since $\tau = 8$ hours and $\ln(2) = 0.6931$ we have

$$\lambda = \frac{0.6931}{8} = 0.0866.$$

If the inoculum consists of sensitive cells only (a common assumption), then

$$S_0 = 8 \times 10^5,$$

$$R_0 = 0.$$

The number of sensitive cells present after 3 days is, therefore, given by Equation 5.5:

$$S(t) = S_0 e^{\lambda t} = 8 \times 10^5 \times e^{0.0866 \times 72} = 4.08 \times 10^8.$$

Assuming resistant cells to grow at the same rate as sensitive cells, the number of resistant cells is given by Equation 5.6:

$$R(72) = R_0 e^{\lambda 72} + \alpha \lambda 72 S_0 e^{\lambda 72}$$

$$= 0 + 1 \times 10^{-7} \times 0.0866 \times 72 \times 4.08 \times 10^8 = 2.54 \times 10^2.$$

That is, there are expected to be approximately 250 resistant cells at the time of treatment.

We may use the two Equations 5.5 and 5.6 to obtain an expression for the overall number of tumour cells, $N(t)$.

$$N(t) = S(t) + R(t) = S_0 e^{\lambda t} + [R_0 e^{\lambda t} + \alpha \lambda t S_0 e^{\lambda t}]$$

$$= [S_0 e^{\lambda t} + R_0 e^{\lambda t}] + \alpha \lambda t S_0 e^{\lambda t} = N_0 e^{\lambda t} + \alpha \lambda t S_0 e^{\lambda t}. \tag{5.7}$$

Equations 5.1 and 5.7 seem to be contradictory when compared in that they provide different expressions for $N(t)$. The reason for this difference is the simplifying assumption made in deriving Equation 5.5 where $[1 - \alpha]$ was replaced by 1. If we do not make this simplification, we obtain slightly different formulae, which when added give Equation 5.1.

In many applications $R_0 = 0$ and the value of α is sufficiently small so that the value of $\alpha \lambda t$ is much less than unity, then

$$N(t) \cong S(t) = S_0 e^{\lambda t}. \tag{5.8}$$

Under these circumstances, the proportion of resistant cells, $R(t)/N(t)$, is approximately equal to Equation 5.6 divided by Equation 5.8:

$$\frac{R(t)}{N(t)} \cong \frac{\alpha \lambda t S_0 e^{\lambda t}}{S_0 e^{\lambda t}} = \alpha \lambda t. \tag{5.9}$$

This final equation demonstrates that the proportion of resistant cells increases linearly as the tumour ages (and grows) so that we would expect older (larger) tumours to be proportionately more resistant.

5.3 General model of tumour growth

An alternative approach is to ignore the time course of growth of the tumour and just use the growth of the tumour as an index (much in the way time is used in the exponential model) of development of the system. This can then be combined with the model of resistance where it is assumed that the likelihood of transitions to resistance are related to tumour growth. In a tumour system where cells neither die nor escape the system, the amount of tumour growth is equal to the number of passages through the cell cycle. We hypothesize that every time a cell moves through the cycle there is a constant probability, α, that the cell becomes resistant and we may then relate this to tumour growth in order to develop formulae for the evolution of resistance. We may formulate these hypotheses mathematically in a way similar to that used in Section 5.2; however, it is not possible to develop differential equations with respect to time since events are not dependent upon time. In this case, we assume that cell divisions are required before transitions to resistance can occur. How do we formulate this? If we are prepared to consider approximating the cell division process, where integer numbers (0, 1, 2, etc.) of cells are added to the overall population, with a smooth process where arbitrarily small fractions of a cell can be added then we may again utilize differential calculus. Let S, R and N represent the sensitive, resistant and total cell compartments of the tumour. We wish to write equations of what happens to the S and R compartments as the overall size N increases; N now replaces t as an index of the overall process, so that we write $S(N)$ and $R(N)$. In this situation we wish to develop equations that will describe the sizes of S and R for any particular value of N. The resulting equations will not describe the growth of the overall population but indicate for a given N what the relative numbers of sensitive and resistant cells are. We assume, as before, that at some particular point (i.e. some size N) we know the number of sensitive (S) and resistant (R) cells. Then we consider what happens when the total number of cells, N, increases to $N + \Delta N$. If we refer to the associated changes in S and R as ΔS and ΔR, respectively, then we have

$$\Delta N = \Delta S + \Delta R, \qquad (5.10)$$

i.e. the increase in the total number is the sum of the increases in the number of sensitive cells and resistant cells. Now ΔR, the increase in the number of resistant cells, consists of the sum of two components, the increase via division of previously existing resistant cells (call this $\Delta R'$) and the influx of new resistant cells converted from sensitivity (call this $\Delta R''$). Therefore, we also have

$$\Delta R = \Delta R' + \Delta R''. \tag{5.11}$$

If resistant and sensitive cells are dividing at the same rate then the rate of increase through division in the resistant cell compartment will equal that in the overall tumour so that

$$\frac{\Delta R'}{R} = \frac{\Delta N}{N},$$

from which we obtain

$$\Delta R' = R\frac{\Delta N}{N}. \tag{5.12}$$

If there is no cell death then the change in the number of cells ΔN equals the number of divisions in the total population. The sensitive cells divide and add both sensitive cells, ΔS, and newly converted resistant cells, $\Delta R''$. The sum $\Delta S + \Delta R''$ is thus equal to the number of sensitive cell divisions. By substituting Equation 5.11 into Equation 5.10 we have,

$$\Delta N = \Delta S + \Delta R' + \Delta R'',$$

so that

$$\Delta S + \Delta R'' = \Delta N - \Delta R'. \tag{5.13}$$

Substituting Equation 5.12 into Equation 5.13 gives an expression for the number of sensitive cell divisions as a function of changes in the overall size of the tumour (ΔN), i.e.

$$\Delta S + \Delta R'' = \Delta N - \Delta R' = \Delta N - R\frac{\Delta N}{N} = \Delta N(1 - R/N). \tag{5.14}$$

A more intuitive explanation of this expression is obtained by noting that $(1 - R/N) = S/N$ equals the proportion of sensitive cells; the formula just says that the number of sensitive cell divisions is equal to the overall number of divisions multiplied by the proportion of sensitive cells in the tumour.

As discussed earlier, we hypothesize that a proportion, α, of sensitive cell divisions convert to resistance at every division. The number of resistant cells created by sensitive cell divisions, $\Delta R''$, is given by α

multiplied by the number of divisions in the sensitive cells, so from Equation 5.14 we obtain

$$\Delta R'' = \alpha(\Delta S + \Delta R'') = \alpha \Delta N(1 - R/N). \qquad (5.15)$$

The increase in the number of resistant cells, ΔR, is obtained by substituting Equations 5.12 and 5.15 into Equation 5.11 to give

$$\begin{aligned} \Delta R = \Delta R' + \Delta R'' &= \Delta N(R/N) + \alpha \Delta N(1 - R/N) \\ &= \alpha \Delta N + \Delta N(1 - \alpha)(R/N). \end{aligned} \qquad (5.16)$$

If we now divide Equation 5.16 through by ΔN and replace the ratio of changes in cell numbers, $(\Delta R/\Delta N)$, by the instantaneous rate of change, dR/dN, then we obtain a differential equation for the number of resistant cells R in terms of the overall number of cells N, i.e.

$$\frac{dR}{dN} = \frac{\Delta R}{\Delta N} = \alpha + (1 - \alpha)(R/N).$$

Solving this equation is quite straightforward so that we obtain the resulting formula for the number of resistant cells in terms of the total number of cells

$$R = N[1 - (1 - R_0/N_0)(N/N_0)^{-\alpha}],$$

where R_0 and N_0 are the sizes of the tumour at some earlier point. If we make the usual assumption that the tumour originated from a single cell that was sensitive then $R_0 = 0$ and $N_0 = 1$. The formula then becomes

$$R = N[1 - N^{-\alpha}]. \qquad (5.17)$$

Accordingly, the proportion of resistant cells, R/N, is given by $(1 - N^{-\alpha})$, from which it is apparent that the proportion of resistant cells increases as the tumour grows. That the proportion is increasing may be seen more readily if we use the approximation $(1 - N^{-\alpha}) \cong \alpha \ln(N)$, which is valid for small values of α and large values of N, so that we get

$$R = \alpha N \ln(N). \qquad (5.18)$$

and the proportion of resistant cells is $\alpha \ln(N)$

We may compare the proportion of resistant cells in the general model to that obtained for the exponential model. If we refer back to Equation 5.9 the formula for the proportion of resistant cells in the exponential growth model, the proportion of resistant cells was $\alpha \lambda t$. If, as usual, the sensitive cells are assumed to form the majority of the tumour, then the total number of cells under the exponential model is given by $N(t) = e^{\lambda t}$ (Equation 5.1) assuming $N_0 = 1$. Substituting this expression into the general expression for the proportion of resistant cells $\alpha \ln(N)$ gives $\alpha \ln(e^{\lambda t}) = \alpha \lambda t$: the same expression as Equation 5.9. The exponential and general models give the same result for the proportion of resistant cells but the exponential model also indicates the size of the tumour as a function of time.

The important difference in the two models is that in the second we make no assumption regarding the exponential growth of the tumour cells. The essential element of both formulae is that they indicate (a) that the *number* of resistant cells *increases* as the overall tumour size increases and (b) that the *proportion* of resistant cells *slowly increases* as the tumour grows. The preceding calculations are based on the random mutation model and it is of some interest to consider what, if any, difference there would be if the directed mutation model was used. The directed mutation model would also predict an increase in the number of resistant cells produced as the tumour size at drug exposure increases. However, the rate of change in the number of resistant cells as tumour size increases is different in the two models so that the directed mutant model would predict that the *proportion* of resistant cells would remain *constant* as the tumour size increases. Unfortunately, the difference in the evolution of the proportion of resistant cells is not a characteristic of the models that may be easily exploited to distinguish between them.

The preceding formulae do not acknowledge the stochastic nature of the resistance process. These formulae provide a way to calculate the *average* number of resistant cells, but as we have already seen in Chapter 4, the actual values in any particular tumour may vary considerably from the average. Also real systems experience alterations in growth conditions that will add to the variation in the numbers of resistant cells in identical tumours. The question, therefore, arises as to whether there is some other quality of resistance, which is more stably measured between tumours, that has some useful interpretation. Such a quantity is the probability of no resistant cells, which we will now discuss.

5.4   Probability of no resistance

When dealing with spontaneous human tumours we deal with a unique occurrence every time. The tumour is composed of cells that inherit an altered form of a person's DNA. Tumours show similarity in behaviour so that it is possible to develop classes within which individual tumours will tend to behave similarly; however, it is important to keep in mind the potential uniqueness of each clinical cancer. The same property exists for passaged animal cancers and *in vitro* tumour systems: different lines display considerable variation in properties and behaviour. The difference is that experimental cancers are also passaged and maintained many times so that it is possible to explore and enumerate the properties of these systems with considerable accuracy providing sufficient resources are available. In this way it is possible to select systems for further study that have interesting or appropriate characteristics. Stability is an important property of an experimental system but one that cannot be assumed in human cancer. An experimenter selecting a system for the study of factors that influence chemotherapy effectiveness would not wish to select one in which chemotherapy was either always or never effective, since such a system would provide little scope for exploration. Therefore, the tendency is to select systems that in their *wild state* display sensitivity to one or more drugs. The relevance of this is that we assume that the wild state in which the experimental tumour is passaged is primarily a drug-sensitive state and it can be eradicated by one or more drugs in some circumstances. Notice there is no requirement that human cancers have this property and a major problem may be that a great number of them do not.

We may characterize a tumour as being in a drug-sensitive state if there are no drug-resistant cells. Conversely it is in a drug-resistant state if there are one or more drug-resistant cells. A tumour converts from a drug-sensitive to a drug-resistant state when one or more drug-resistant cells come into being. Calculating the average number of resistant cells, using the formulae of the previous section, does not give much insight into the transition between sensitivity and resistance since the average is almost always greater than zero and increases continuously without any jumps marking the creation of individual cells. However, a quantity that can be calculated is the probability, P_0, that there are no resistant cells present to the drug under consideration. The probability will be viewed as a function of time or tumour size and will be written as $P_0(t)$ or $P_0(N)$, respectively. Initially, we will derive an expression for P_0 based on the general model of growth that will apply to the exponential model as a special case.

Derivation of a formula for $P_0(N)$ is based upon the simple observation that there will be no resistant cells if, and only if, there are none created. The distribution of the number of resistant cells created from sensitive cells has a Poisson distribution with parameter equal to the mean number created (see Equation 2.5, p. 40). The mean number created is equal to the mean number of transitions from sensitivity to resistance and not to the number of resistant cells, which also includes cells deriving from the division of pre-existing resistant cells. Here we will assume, as before, that α represents the proportion of divisions of sensitive cells that produces a new resistant cell. The mean number of new resistant cells created from sensitive cells is α multiplied by the number of sensitive cell divisions. If at the beginning, the tumour consists of N_0 cells and at some later time it consists of N cells then there will have been $N - N_0$ total divisions since each division adds one cell (assuming no cell loss or death). The mean number, μ, of new resistant cells created is given by

$$\mu = \alpha(N - N_0).$$

The probability of a zero count in a Poisson distribution with mean μ is given by $e^{-\mu}$ (see Equation 4.6), so the probability of no resistant cells at size N ($P_0(N)$), is given by

$$P_0(N) = e^{-\alpha(N-N_0)}. \tag{5.19}$$

When this formula is applied to human cancer, which is assumed to grow from a single cell origin, it is common to set $N_0 = 1$ so that

$$P_0(t) = e^{-\alpha(N-1)}. \tag{5.20}$$

In a number of contexts $P_0(N)$ has been referred to as the *probability of cure*, since it represents the maximum proportion of cures that can be achieved by the application of the drug under consideration. The idea being that, at least in principle, all drug-sensitive cells can be destroyed by the drug and that one or more pre-existing resistant cells will lead to eventual regrowth of the tumour in a drug-resistant state. The actual proportion of cures depends upon the way in which the drug is administered and the rate of growth of the tumour. The formula would be accurate if all drug-sensitive cells were eliminated at the time of first drug application. For all but the smallest tumours this will not be true and some sensitive cells will survive and grow. This growth has the potential to produce resistance so that Equation 5.20 is only an approximation.

The more rapid the reduction in size of the tumour and the less opportunity for regrowth the better will be the agreement between $P_0(N)$ and the observed proportion of cures.

Plots of $P_0(N)$, as a function of the tumour size, N, (Equation 5.20) are given in Fig. 5.2 for different values of α. We see immediately the characteristic sigmoid shape of each plot of $P_0(N)$, which has the same 'shape' for all values of α. Each plot appears to be the same except that they are translated horizontally for different values of α. We anticipate this from Equation 5.20 for $P_0(N)$, since if $N \gg 1$ then $N - 1 \cong N$, and

$$P_0(N) \cong e^{-\alpha N}. \tag{5.21}$$

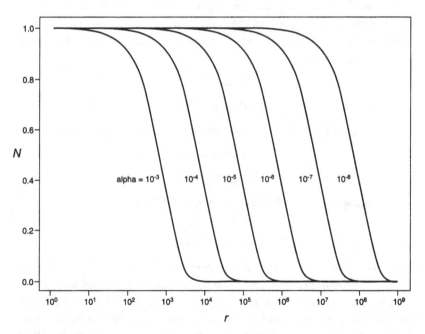

Fig. 5.2. Plot of the probability of no resistant cells, $P_0(N)$, as a function of the tumour size, N, and the transition rate, α. The tumour size, N, is displayed on a logarithmic scale. It can be seen that the probability starts at unity, by assumption, and declines to 0, following a profile that is determined by the value of the product αN, as is evident from the approximate formula $P_0(n) \cong \exp(-\alpha N)$. It can be seen that the value of $P_0(N)$, for each value of α, changes from a high to low value over a region representing the same sized shift in the abscissa. This implies that the probability changes in the same way for the same proportionate increase in growth for each value of α.

In Equation 5.21 it is only the product αN that influences $P_0(N)$, so that decreasing the value of α 10-fold has exactly the same effect as a 10-fold decrease in the tumour size N. Other things being equal, selection of a drug with a lower value of α will provide an equivalent therapeutic outcome in a larger tumour. Of course it must be kept in mind that when comparing real drugs 'other things are seldom equal'.

We may express the similarity of the plots of $P_0(N)$ for different values of α in another way. Consider what happens in a growing tumour as N increases. At first $P_0(N)$ is close to unity and remains this way until the tumour size, N, is sufficiently large that $P_0(N)$ starts to decline rapidly (this happens when N is large enough that $\alpha N > 0.1$). The plot subsequently reaches a plateau at zero when N is sufficiently large. What change in N is required to take $P_0(N)$ from a high value to a low value? If we let P_H represent the high value and P_L represent the low value and N_H and N_L represent the respective tumour sizes, then from Equation 5.21 we have

$$P_H = e^{-\alpha N_H}$$
$$P_L = e^{-\alpha N_L}.$$

If we then take logarithms (to the base e) of these equations we obtain

$$\ln(P_H) = -\alpha N_H$$
$$\ln(P_L) = -\alpha N_L$$

Finally taking the ratio of these last two equations gives

$$\frac{\ln(P_H)}{\ln(P_L)} = \frac{N_H}{N_L} \tag{5.22}$$

Note that Equation 5.22 does not depend on the value of α, so that the change in probability will occur during the same fractional increase in the tumour size N_H/N_L. This is not to say that N_H and N_L do not depend upon α but that their ratio is the same for any value of α. We may characterize this as saying that every tumour type moves from a high probability to a low probability of resistance during the same proportionate increase in size, no matter what the value of α, as long as the tumour starts in a drug-sensitive state. What α does is to determine when, in the history of the tumour, this change is likely to occur. When we refer in this discussion to a tumour type, we are referring to the process of resistance development in a class of homogeneous tumours. In any single tumour where the model is valid, it actually undergoes a virtually instantaneous transformation from sensitivity to resistance with the appearance of the first resistant cell.

The preceding relationship has an even easier interpretation when the tumour grows exponentially. Under exponential growth the size at time t is given by,

$$N(t) = N_0 e^{\lambda t}.$$

Now if we designate t_H as the time at which the tumour is size N_H and t_L the time at which it is size N_L, then the above equation indicates

$$N_H = N_0 e^{\lambda t_H}$$
$$N_L = N_0 e^{\lambda t_L}.$$

If we take the ratio of N_H to N_L, then we obtain

$$\frac{N_H}{N_L} = \frac{N_0 e^{\lambda t_H}}{N_0 e^{\lambda t_L}} = e^{\lambda(t_H - t_L)}$$

Now if we now use Equation 5.22 with the above equation we have

$$\frac{\ln(P_H)}{\ln(P_L)} = \frac{N_H}{N_L} = e^{\lambda(t_H - t_L)}.$$

This equation says that the transition from a low probability of resistance to a high probability of resistance occurs over an interval of time, $t_H - t_L$ which does not depend on the value of α and does depend on the growth rate λ of the tumour. This rather simple relationship provides a powerful tool for examining experimental assessments of resistance and implies the existence of invariants, such as the length of the interval $t_H - t_L$ in a single tumour system treated with different drugs. Of course this deduction is only true in tumour systems that have the same characteristics as assumed in the development of this mathematical model.

It is worthwhile considering what effects one would expect under the directed model compared with the random model, which has been employed up to now. The short answer is that there is very little difference in the predictions for $P_0(t)$ which would be obtained using either model: it is more a matter of expressing what the results say. Under the directed mutation model, tumours do not continuously convert from sensitivity to resistance but remain sensitive until exposure to the drug. At exposure the probability that none are converted to resistance is given by Equation 5.21 with α replaced by ρ. For the directed model this formula is again an approximation but the nature of the approximation is somewhat different. For the directed model, it is the remaining number of sensitive cells at any subsequent drug treatment and not the regrowth between drug treatments, as for the random mutation model. Again (Section 5.3) the random and directed models result in similar predictions for measurable characteristics of a tumour system (the probability of cure).

5.5   Experimental evidence

The extreme variability between individual tumours in clinical cancer prevent simple testing of the relationships developed in this chapter. Experimental tumour systems provide a far greater opportunity for verification, since many factors that affect outcome have been studied and characterized. As discussed in Chapter 2, Skipper and his colleagues have made major strides in characterizing determinants of outcome and produced a vast amount of valuable data. In the discussion of *in vivo* fluctuation tests in Chapter 4, it was noted that different measures of therapeutic outcome are not all equally useful in providing sensitive measures of resistance endpoints. Obviously, median survival time (the time until 50% of the animals have died) is only useful when more than 50% will die. Even when evaluable, the median survival time may be only modestly affected by differences as large as 10-fold in the value of α, so that measurement of this statistic may not be ideal for exploring the resistance process.[†] The residual tumour burden after treatment is very dependent upon the value of α, as may be seen from Equation 5.17. However, it can be difficult to measure since the number of tumour cells may be below the level of clinical measurement. It is possible to allow the tumour to grow to a fixed measurable size and then

---

[†] This arises because most treatments undergoing evaluation in such systems are at least moderately effective against sensitive cells. Such treatment results in substantial tumour reduction, which will eventually reach its limiting effect when only resistant cells remain. The size of the remainder is determined by α, and the remainder will tend to be small since the treatment is effective. A ten-fold decrease or increase in the remainder will not make a great difference to the survival time since this time consists mostly of the regrowth period required for the tumour to clinically re-emerge and subsequently cause the animal's death. For example, if death occurs at 10^8 cells, it will take approximately 20 doubling times to death if 100 cells remain postchemotherapy. If 1000 cells remain it will require approximately 17 doubling periods. A 10-fold change in the post-treatment tumour burden (which would result if α were 10 times as large) results in only a 15% reduction in the median survival time.

use knowledge of the tumour growth characteristics to estimate the post-treatment disease burden. The main problem with this measurement is the great variability between tumours treated in an identical fashion. Of course this is a major consequence of the random mutation theory and is the basis of the fluctuation test.

A convenient and easily measured quantity is the fraction of surviving animals (for *in vivo* experiments) or the proportion of colonies which regrow (for *in vitro* experiments). These quantities are exactly those given by the probability of cure function, $P_0(N)$. It is not the purpose of this chapter to examine exhaustively the wealth of experimental data available; however, an example is reproduced in Table 5.1.

Table 5.1 represents data on the treatment of almost 600 mice using a single drug, ara-C. The information has been compiled from a number of clinical trials carried out by Skipper and colleagues using intraperitoneally (i.p.) and intravenously (i.v.) implanted L1210 leukaemia cells. The data were collected from experiments in which a fixed number (usually between 100 and 1000) of leukaemia cells were directly implanted into an animal. The growth of the tumour is known to be regular, for inocula in this range, and the size at any later time can be accurately estimated from the initial innoculum size and the elapsed time. Previous experimentation had demonstrated that the implantation of a single leukaemia cell was sufficient to lead to death of the animal within 45 days; similarly, animals with the leukaemia surviving 45 days post-treatment were free of residual disease. The data presented in Table 5.1 give the number of 45-day survivors.

The drug ara-C is especially active against cells in the S phase of the cell cycle and hence its effect is limited by the proportion of cells in this phase during treatment. This drug is administered at doses far below the LD_{10} (the dose at which 10% of the treated animals would die of toxicity) since larger doses have no greater tumoricidal effect (as expected for a phase-specific drug (Chapter 2)). The data reported consist of the observed outcome in relation to the number of courses of treatment (Table 5.1). Where multiple courses were given there was a period of 3 days of no treatment between each consecutive course.

A number of patterns can be identified in the data. Firstly, within each group of experiments where the same number of courses were given we notice an inverse relationship between the size of the tumour when treatment began and the proportion of animals cured. Secondly, for tumours having the same size at initial treatment the proportion of

Table 5.1. *Results of treatment with ara-C of DBA mice implanted with the experimental L1210 mouse leukaemia*

Schedule:[a] number of courses	Size at treatment $N(t)$	Number of animals treated	Number of survivors[b]	Proportion cured
1	8×10^6	10	0	0.00
	8×10^5	60	2	0.03
	8×10^4	20	11	0.55
2	8×10^7	20	0	0.00
	8×10^6	40	3	0.08
	8×10^5	19	11	0.58
3	8×10^6	9	3	0.33
	8×10^5	30	25	0.83
4	8×10^7	59	0	0.00
	8×10^6	80	25	0.31
	8×10^5	215	187	0.87
	8×10^4	30	30	1.00

[a] Each course consisted of a dose of 15 mg/kg body weight every 3 hours for eight doses.
[b] Animals surviving 45 days post-treatment were free of residual disease.

cures increases with number of courses given, although this relationship is not so regular as the first. How do these observations accord with the random mutation model? Before presenting the results of a formal analysis we can consider what factors should influence the observed outcomes.

1. If we do not give sufficient drug, that is enough courses, the sensitive cells will not be eliminated and the leukaemia will regrow and kill the animal irrespective of whether there are resistant cells present.
2. We are less likely to give sufficient drug when the tumour load at first treatment is greater because we have more cells to eliminate.
3. Smaller tumours are less likely to have resistant cells present so that when sufficient drug is given to eliminate the sensitive cells they are more likely to be eradicated than larger tumours.
4. Larger tumours are more likely to have resistant cells; as a result they are less likely to show any relationship between the number of courses and the cure rate.

Table 5.1 displays exactly the anticipated relationships. One course eradicates 55% of tumours consisting of 8×10^4 cells at first treatment, whereas four courses eradicates 100%, suggesting that there are unlikely to be resistant cells present but that one course is insufficient to eliminate the sensitive cells. Four courses eradicate 87% of tumours of initial size 8×10^5 where three courses cures a similar proportion, suggesting that the sensitive cells have been eliminated after three courses and further treatment is ineffective. However, the observation that neither of these observed cure rates are 100% suggests that resistant cells are present. We would, therefore, anticipate that further increases in the initial size at first treatment would produce a rapid change in the proportion of cures since we know that $P_0(N)$ is in a portion of the sigmoid curve where it changes rapidly (Fig. 5.2). We would also predict that since it took three courses to eliminate all the sensitive cells in a tumour of size 8×10^5 it would take at least three courses to eliminate the sensitive cells in a tumour of 8×10^6; tumours not cured with two or less courses would represent resistance plus a failure to eliminate sensitive cells. We see exactly the anticipated pattern in Table 5.1. The proportion of cures for three and four courses are the same (33% and 31%, respectively) and lower than the cure rate achieved by the same number of courses when the tumour size was smaller. Also the proportion cured at 8×10^6 is less for two courses (8%) and even less for one course (0%), indicating that sensitive cells are also causing treatment failure. Finally, treatment of tumours of size 8×10^7 produces no cures even for four courses, indicating that resistance is almost certainly present and treatment can only delay death not prevent it.

The preceding 'explanation' of the data provides a persuasive case for drug resistance-mediated treatment failure along the lines proposed earlier in the chapter. A more rigorous analysis can made by statistically fitting the equations derived to the observed data. Since the drug is only given at a single dosage level it is not necessary to model the dose response function of the sensitive cells. We assumed that each cycle in a course caused the same log kill amongst sensitive cells and estimated the magnitude of that log kill from the data. The tumour was assumed to grow exponentially with an 8 hour doubling time, as had been previously reported. A more general formulation of the random mutation model was fitted to the data, which permitted the parameter α to vary between experiments. This was done to provide a test of validity of the model used. The theory required to carry out such an analysis is described elsewhere (Coldman and Goldie, 1988).

Table 5.2. *Observed and predicted cure proportions for the L1210 leukaemia treated with ara-C*

Schedule:[a] number of courses	Size at treatment $N(t)$	Observed proportion cured	95% confidence interval	Predicted proportion cured
1	8×10^6	0.00	0.00, 0.31	0.00
	8×10^5	0.03	0.00, 0.12	0.02
	8×10^4	0.55	0.32, 0.77	0.68
2	8×10^7	0.00	0.00, 0.17	0.00
	8×10^6	0.08	0.02, 0.21	0.22
	8×10^5	0.58	0.33, 0.80	0.86
3	8×10^6	0.33	0.07, 0.70	0.22
	8×10^5	0.83	0.65, 0.94	0.86
4	8×10^7	0.00	0.00, 0.06	0.00
	8×10^6	0.31	0.21, 0.43	0.22
	8×10^5	0.87	0.82, 0.91	0.86
	8×10^4	1.00	0.88, 1.00	0.99

[a]Each course consisted of a dose of 15 mg/kg body weight every 3 hours for eight doses.

The process of fitting these models is somewhat complicated and only the results of the analysis are presented in Table 5.2. Agreement between the theory and experimental results is not perfect but is certainly reasonable, and all but one cure rate predicted by using the random mutation model lies within the 95% confidence interval of the data. Each cycle of therapy was found to kill 81% of sensitive cells and it was the rapid repopulation rate of the tumour that required the use of multiple courses. The random mutation parameter α was estimated as 1.8×10^{-7}. The model fitted the data well and there was no evidence of any variation in the parameter. It must be kept in mind that animals may die from causes other than leukaemia so that the proportion surviving is likely to underestimate the proportion in which the disease was eradicated.

Table 5.3 gives the results of another series of experiments, in which the L1210 leukaemia was treated with the drug cyclophosphamide. Data on the action of cyclophosphamide suggest that it is active in all phases of the cell cycle. In these experiments, varying doses were administered in a single treatment and the resulting cures observed in the same way as for the ara-C data. This table also contains separate data on two modes

Table 5.3. *Results of treatment with cyclophosphamide of DBA mice implanted either intravenously or intraperitoneally with the experimental L1210 mouse leukaemia*

Dose (mg/kg)	Size at treatment (N(t))	Intraperitoneal implantation			Intravenous implantation		
		No. animals treated	No. survivors	Proportion cured	No. animals treated	No. survivors	Proportion cured
300	8×10^7	94	7	0.07	80	4	0.05
	8×10^6	148	60	0.41	30	10	0.33
	8×10^5	39	30	0.77	20	14	0.70
250	8×10^7	–	–	–	66	1	0.02
	8×10^6	–	–	–	30	3	0.10
	8×10^5	–	–	–	30	17	0.57
230	8×10^6	50	7	0.14	–	–	–
	8×10^5	40	10	0.25	–	–	–
	8×10^4	50	41	0.82	–	–	–
200	8×10^7	109	3	0.03	60	0	0.00
	8×10^6	160	11	0.07	40	3	0.08
	8×10^5	60	11	0.18	10	0	0.00
	8×10^4	10	8	0.80	–	–	–
	8×10^3	10	10	1.00	–	–	–
150	8×10^7	30	0	0.00	245	0	0.00
	8×10^6	19	0	0.00	60	0	0.00
	8×10^5	20	1	0.05	50	3	0.06
100	8×10^7	10	0	0.00	130	0	0.00
	8×10^6	20	0	0.00	30	0	0.00
	8×10^5	144	0	0.00	20	0	0.00

of implantation of the tumour: intraperitoneally and intravenously. Very similar patterns are observed in these data to that seen in the response of the same tumour to ara-C. If the tumour is too large then resistance seems certain and cure is not achieved with any of the doses. If the dose is too small when the tumour is small, then again cure will not be achieved because the sensitive cells were not eliminated.

As in the case with ara-C, we may undertake a more rigorous analysis of statistically fitting the formulae for the probability of cure to the data. Since varying doses are given in a single injection, rather than a constant dose repeatedly administered as for the ara-C data, it is necessary to fit a dose response function to the cell kill achieved by drug on the sensitive cells. In this case we have used the log kill law as described in Section 1.9. Again a more general random mutation resistance model was used, which permitted the parameter α to vary between experiments and by route of implantation of the tumour. If the random mutation model is correct than we would not expect α to vary by route of implantation.

The fitted probabilities are given in Table 5.4. The fit of the model to these data is not as good as for the ara-C experiments. Examination of the pattern of fit suggests that this may be owing to inaccuracy in the assumed kill function for the sensitive cells. It appears that the log kill law is not accurate over the full range of doses, with lesser effects than predicted at higher doses. This phenomenon was noted by Bruce and co-workers who observed a plateauing of cyclophosphamide effect at very high log kills (six logs) (Valeriote, Bruce and Meeker, 1968). The estimated values implied that the log kill associated with 200 mg/kg was approximately seven logs. Because of the statistical process of fitting, this manifests itself as overestimation of the efficacy at high doses and underestimation at low doses. Since resistance is the major reason for incurability at the higher doses, we tend to see this overestimation more in the middle range of doses. The mutation parameter was estimated to be 1.0×10^{-7}. The estimated mutation rate did not vary with the route of administration, supporting the notion that the reason for the patterns of response to treatment in these data is a resistance phenomenon of the type postulated. Using a curvilinear dose response model improves the fit but does not substantially affect the preceding results.

The kind of analysis presented here has been done fairly infrequently so there is not a large body of analytical evidence that can be examined. However, the pattern which emerges from examination of many of the experimental data available is similar to that given in the two examples

Table 5.4. *Results of treatment with cyclophosphamide of DBA mice implanted either intravenously or intraperitoneally with the experimental L1210 mouse leukaemia*

Dose (mg/kg)	Size at treatment ($N(t)$)	Intraperitoneal implantation			Intravenous implantation		
		Observed proportion cured	95% confidence interval	Predicted proportion cured	Observed proportion cured	95% confidence interval	Predicted proportion cured
300	8×10^7	0.07	0.03, 0.15	0.00	0.05	0.00, 0.12	0.00
	8×10^6	0.41	0.33, 0.49	0.44	0.33	0.17, 0.53	0.43
	8×10^5	0.77	0.61, 0.89	0.92	0.70	0.46, 0.88	0.92
250	8×10^7	–	–	–	0.02	0.00, 0.08	0.00
	8×10^6	–	–	–	0.10	0.02, 0.27	0.42
	8×10^5	–	–	–	0.57	0.37, 0.75	0.92
230	8×10^6	0.14	0.06, 0.27	0.39	–	–	–
	8×10^5	0.25	0.13, 0.41	0.91	–	–	–
	8×10^4	0.82	0.68, 0.91	0.99	–	–	–
200	8×10^7	0.03	0.00, 0.08	0.00	0.00	0.00, 0.06	0.00
	8×10^6	0.07	0.00, 0.12	0.15	0.08	0.02, 0.21	0.18
	8×10^5	0.18	0.10, 0.30	0.82	0.00	0.00, 0.31	0.84
	8×10^4	0.80	0.44, 0.97	0.98	–	–	–
	8×10^3	1.00	0.69, 1.00	1.00	–	–	–
150	8×10^7	0.00	0.00, 0.12	0.00	0.00	0.00, 0.01	0.00
	8×10^6	0.00	0.00, 0.18	0.00	0.00	0.00, 0.06	0.00
	8×10^5	0.05	0.00, 0.25	0.00	0.06	0.00, 0.17	0.01
100	8×10^7	0.00	0.00, 0.31	0.00	0.00	0.00, 0.03	0.00
	8×10^6	0.00	0.00, 0.17	0.00	0.00	0.00, 0.12	0.00
	8×10^5	0.00	0.00, 0.04	0.00	0.00	0.00, 0.17	0.00

above. It would appear that resistance, of the form developed here, seems a major contributor to the failure of cancer chemotherapy in experimental systems.

5.6   Summary and conclusions

In this chapter a mathematical formulation of the random mutation model has been developed and built around simple models for tumour growth. It was shown that the form of the growth curve was not critical as long as there was no cell loss or death. It was demonstrated that both the number and the proportion of resistant cells increase as the tumour grows. The random mutation rate parameter, α, was shown to control the overall number of resistant cells. A quantity, the probability of no resistant cells (P_0) was identified as a critical measure of the behaviour of the tumour in that it described the conversion of the tumour from a curable to an incurable state by the drug. The value of P_0 was shown to depend on α but it was found that all types of tumour originating in a drug-sensitive state would pass through a region of growth, of constant relative size, where they went from a low to a high probability of containing drug-resistant cells. Finally it was shown how predictions using this model yielded reasonable explanations of the patterns seen in some experimental data.

References

Coldman, A.J. and Goldie, J.H. (1988). The effect of tumor heterogeneity on the development of resistance to anti-cancer agents and its impliction for neo-adjuvant chemotherapy. In *Proc. 2nd Int. Congr. Neo-Adjuvant Chemotherapy*, Paris, 19–21 February, pp. 37–41. John Libbey Eurotext.

Valeriote, F.A., Bruce, W.R. and Meeker, B.E. (1968). Synergistic action of cyclophosphamide and 1,3-bis(2-chloroethyl)-1-nitrosourea on a transplanted murine lymphoma. *J. Natl. Cancer Inst.*, 40: 936–944.

Further reading

Goldie, J.H. and Coldman, A.J. (1979). A mathematic model for relating the drug sensitivity of tumours to their spontaneous mutation rate. *Cancer Treat. Rep.*, 63: 1727–1733.

Skipper, H.E., Schabel, F.M. and Wilcox, W.S. (1975). Experimental evaluation of potential anti-cancer agents, XIV; further study of certain basic concepts underlying chemotherapy of leukemia. *Cancer Chemother. Rep.*, 45: 5–28.

Skipper, H.E., Schabel, F.M. and Lloyd, H.H. (1979). Dose response and tumour cell repopulation rate in chemotherapeutic trials. In *Advances in Cancer Chemotherapy*, Vol. 1, ed. A. Rozownki, pp. 205–253. Marcel Dekker, New York.

Steel, G.G. (1977). *Growth Kinetics of Tumours*. Clarendon Press, Oxford.

6

Extensions of the random mutation model for drug resistance

6.1 Introduction

We are coming to what some readers may find to be the most difficult section of the book because we will attempt to synthesize a number of the mathematical developments we have described previously into a more complex model that is intended to conform more closely to the behaviour of clinical malignancies. The most important elements in this synthesis will be the basic random mutation model of resistance (Chapters 4 and 5) and the stem cell model of tumour growth (Chapter 2). We will describe in more detail the birth/death processes that were introduced in Chapter 2 and indicate how they impact on the issue of drug resistance and the more general question of tumour heterogeneity.

It should be kept in mind that birth/death events are more than just convenient mathematical abstractions for they can provide a mathematical description of the effects of molecular processes that regulate movement through the cell cycle or signal differentiation and apoptosis.

In Chapter 5 we introduced and discussed the random mutation model for resistance to an anticancer drug. This model predicted that tumours which start sensitive would, as they grow, convert to drug resistance by the spontaneous evolution of drug-resistant cells whose population expands at a rate that exceeds that of the tumour as a whole. This model was developed within a framework in which cells divide with unlimited potential (stem cells) forming new stem cells at each expansion. Comparison with data from *in vivo* tumour systems showed that this model accurately simulated and explained the pattern of animal survival seen in some experiments. We also discussed how the directed mutation model makes many similar predictions regarding the pattern of resistance which would be seen in most experiments.

148

In this chapter, we propose to extend the somatic mutation model for resistance and the stem cell model of growth in a number of fundamental ways. We will do this by relaxing some of the assumptions we previously used in these models and expanding the states which a cell can occupy. To do this rigorously would involve considerable mathematical development. Rather than present this theory we will try to provide motivation for the results of such a mathematical development.

One of the great benefits of mathematical development is that it often causes the explicit statement of assumptions that can otherwise be overlooked, especially by those most familiar with the problem. At this point it is instructive to review the assumptions we have made in the mathematical development presented in Chapters 4 and 5. (Undoubtedly the reader will discover some we have made but not included in the list.)

1. Tumour cells divide continuously producing further cells with unlimited growth potential.
2. We only consider resistance to a single drug.
3. Cells may be classified into one of two states, sensitive or resistant, with respect to a single drug.
4. Sensitive cells have a fixed probability of survival after administration of a drug that does not vary with their location within the tumour.
5. All sensitive cells behave in the same way.
6. Resistant cells survive administration of the drug with probability one.
7. Resistant and sensitive cells divide at the same rate.
8. A new resistant cell is created with constant probability, α, at each division of a sensitive cell.
9. Resistant cells remain resistant forever and do not revert to sensitivity.
10 The progenitor tumour cell is in a drug-sensitive state (probably true for some drugs but may not (and almost certainly will not) be true for *all* drugs).

One could attempt to relax all of these assumptions, in specific ways, and determine the resulting effect on the growth of the tumour and the distribution of resistant cells. Although this may be of some mathematical interest we will only be interested in examining those which may influence the manifestation and distribution of drug resistance. As has been discussed in other chapters, although some experimental tumours may appear to consist of homogeneous collections of cells with unlimited growth potential, many do not, and there is considerable evidence that most clinical cancer does not. The first 'assumption' we will examine and modify is number (1).

6.2   Compartment model for tumour growth

The compartment model for tumour growth was first developed by Bush and colleagues at the Ontario Cancer Institute (Bush and Hill, 1975; Chapter 2) and postulates that cells may be classified into one of three categories based upon their growth behaviour: (a) stem cells, (b) transitional cells and (c) end cells. Stem cells are capable of potentially unlimited growth and divide to form either two new stem cells or two transitional cells. Newly created transitional cells are capable of a fixed number of divisions and upon division form further transitional cells, which have less capacity to divide than their ancestor. The terminal divisional stage of the transitional cells is referred to as end cells and comprises cells that have no further capacity to divide. Although end cells may theoretically persist indefinitely, it is likely that they have a limited life span and soon undergo apoptosis. The compartment model is patterned after the growth of the haematopoietic system. In a perfectly regulated system the only mechanism of cell death may be from end cell decay; however, in rapidly growing tumour systems, stem and transitional cells may be eliminated in a variety of ways along the pathway of differentiation.

The compartment model of tumour growth predicts different patterns of tumour behaviour from pure stem cell models. Most importantly, and obviously, it implies that not all cells are capable of new tumour creation so that, for *in vivo* experimental tumours, serial maintenance will involve re-implantation of large numbers of cells in order to guarantee the inclusion of stem cells unless they can be morphologically identified. It also implies that treatment need not eliminate all cells to be successful but only that proportion which have stem cell capacity. In Chapter 2 the probability that a stem cell would divide to form two new stem cells was termed the renewal probability, P, and it was shown how, if this probability was constant, the growth rate of the stem cell compartment was slowed. Also the probability that the line originating from a single stem cell would disappear, the extinction probability, was also calculated and shown to depend on P. An interesting property of the compartment model is that if all its parameters are constant (they do not vary with the age or size of the tumour) as the tumour grows the three cell types reach a dynamic equilibrium where they maintain a constant proportion of cells within the tumour. As a consequence of this, all compartments grow at the same relative rate in this equilibrium stage and this rate of growth is equal to the overall growth rate of the tumour. Because the stem cell compartment is the only compartment not requiring the input of cells from another compartment, it behaves as the engine of growth of the tumour; it is the growth of the stem cell compartment that regulates the overall growth of the tumour.

Even though the stem cells behave as the tumour engine they do not necessarily form a large bulk of the overall tumour size. Obviously the 'mix' of cells changes as the tumour ages. The first cell must be a stem cell, so that the original tumour is 100% stem cell. Subsequently some stem cell divisions result in the creation of transitional cells, which continue dividing. In the initial stages the proportion of various types of cell will be constantly changing since the random result of each single division will be influential. Eventually an equilibrium will be reached[†] in which *the law of large numbers*[‡] becomes applicable and the various compartments settle down to a fixed relationship with respect to one another. The formulae governing the behaviour of the tumour in the equilibrium situation is complex and can only be summarized here.

1. The growth of the stem cell compartment and the total tumour is exponential.
2. The growth rate is $[\ln 2 + \ln P]$ (λ in Equation 5.1, p. 123), on a scale where unity is the interdivision time of the stem cells.
3. The proportion of stem cells in the tumour declines as the renewal probability decreases.

[†] There are actually two equilibria: one in which the tumour continues to grow and one in which it dies and disappears. Now, as pointed out, the stem cells maintain tumour growth so the tumour will die if, and only if, the stem cell line dies. The stem cell line started from a single stem cell so that this probability is equal to what we have previously called the *extinction probability*. Therefore, a proportion, given by the extinction probability, of newly created tumours will die and we will only 'see' the remaining proportion that go on to form viable tumours.

[‡] Laws of large numbers are theorems in probability that relate to the behaviour of the average of observations on many objects (in this case cells) which have identical characteristics. When there are sufficient stem cells, the observed proportion of divisions that result in new stem cells is very close to that which is expected, i.e. P. Then since the overall tumour growth is governed by that of the stem cells everything else follows.

4. The proportion of stem cells decreases as the number of divisions that can be made by the transitional cells increases. (Actually the proportion of stem cells is proportional to P^n where P is the renewal probability and n is the number of potential divisions of each newly created transitional cell.)

What happens when we try to integrate the random mutation model of resistance with this growth model? Firstly, since nonstem cells have only limited growth potential they are unlikely to influence the long-term outcome of treatment. This result does not follow mathematically from the nature of the process but from the likely values of the parameters involved. If transitional cells can only divide a fixed number of times, and this number is not too large, then a single or a few transitional cells will not be able to divide sufficiently to form a large enough tumour to cause clinical disease or death. If, however, a transitional cell was able to divide sufficiently to do this, then we may care to think of it as an 'honorary' stem cell and not a transitional cell. Whether resistance is rare or widespread amongst transitional cells will not influence long-term outcome of treatment. Of course this is not to say that the presence of widespread resistance among such cells will not be a potent determinant of the short-term outcome of treatment, as transitional cells may well constitute the bulk of the tumour. Therefore, in considering long-term treatment outcomes, 'cures', we need only consider what is going on in the stem cell compartment. Secondly, the appearance of a resistant cell in the stem cell compartment does not necessarily imply that the tumour cannot be cured. The resistant cells may spontaneously become extinct in the way any single stem cell lineage may become extinct, by having progeny that lose stem cell capacity.

It would, therefore, seem that using a compartment model for tumour growth rather than a pure stem cell model would imply, other things being equal, that the likelihood of resistance was reduced, since (a) the overall number of stem cells is reduced and only resistant stem cells will influence long-term outcome and (b) stem cells lines are no longer immortal with certainty so that spontaneously arising resistance may spontaneously disappear. However these two effects are not the only ones that influence events and more subtle aspects of the process act to counterbalance them. One such effect will be illustrated in the following example.

Example 6.1

Consider a selection model in which drug resistance spontaneously arises at a common rate in two different tumour systems. The first system is a pure stem cell system (renewal probability $P = 1.0$) and the second is a compartment model with renewal probability 0.55. Each tumour system is grown until there are 1000 stem cells. In the pure stem cell model this will take about 10 interdivision times since $2^{10} = 1024 \cong 1000$. In the compartment model, each division of a stem cell produces, on average, $2P$ stem cells. Two stem cells are produced with probability P and two transitional cells with probability $(1 - P)$. To create 1000 stem cells from a single stem cell will require, on average, just over 72 divisions, since $(2 \times 0.55)^{72} = (1.1)^{72} = 955.6 \cong 1000$. If we consider the age of each stem cell to be measured by the number of divisions to trace back until there was a single stem cell, then each stem cell in the compartment model has a much greater age than a corresponding cell in the pure stem cell system (72 versus 10).

We recall from Chapter 5 that the probability of resistance arising, α, is formulated as a rate of creation per division. The stem cells present in the system where $P = 0.55$ are much 'older' than for the $P = 1$ system. The likelihood that resistance has arisen is much higher, about seven fold (72/10), in each stem cell among the 1000 in the compartment model than in the pure stem cell system. Notice that we are still considering that the acquisition of resistance by a stem cell is completely random and the same in the tumour systems with different values of P. The seemingly 'intuitive' notion that since resistant and sensitive cells are equally likely to go extinct there will be no effect of the overall number of resistant cells is incorrect.

It is the total number of divisions the system has undergone that influences the likelihood of resistance and not the number of cells per se. In the pure stem cell it just happens that the total number of divisions and the number of cells are generally equal. Although Example 6.1 provides an intuitive explanation as to why the proportion of resistant cells would be elevated amongst stem cells in a compartment model compared with a pure stem cell model it does not indicate by how much. This problem proves to be not too complex mathematically since one has to modify the equations of Chapter 5 only slightly.

In Chapter 5 we wrote that for the exponential growth model new resistant cells are arising via transformation at rate

$$\alpha \lambda S(t).$$

(See discussion leading to Equation 5.2, p. 123.) In that case $S(t)$ and $R(t)$ represented the number of sensitive and resistant cells in the whole tumour. Now we will use them to represent the number of sensitive and resistant stem cells. In Section 5.2, α was viewed as a rate per cell division and it was shown that, when growth is exponential, you can convert between the rate per division and the rate per unit time by multiplying the former by the growth rate (λ) of the tumour cell population. When stem cells undergo differentiation, not every division results in an increase in the stem cell population and this simple relationship no longer holds. An appropriate relationship can be derived as follows.

As noted above, in the equilibrium stage of the compartment model the net growth rate of the stem cells equals the growth rate of the overall tumour. Let us call a division of a stem cell to form two stem cells a birth (since it adds a new stem cell) and designate that it happens at rate (per unit time) b. Similarly, a division of a stem cell to form two transitional cells will be called a death (since a stem cell is lost) and the rate of this event can be designated d. The overall growth rate of the stem cells, and, therefore, the whole tumour, is given by the difference in these rates, i.e. $\lambda = b - d$. In Chapter 2 we considered the possibility of stem cell divisions resulting in nonstem cells by the specification of the renewal probability P. What is the relationship of P to b and d? The overall rate of stem cell division is given by $b + d$ and the rate resulting in stem cell additions is b. Thus a proportion $b/(b + d)$ results in stem cell births, which is nothing else than the renewal probability $P = b/(b + d)$. As b is the rate at which new stem cells are being created, αb is the rate at which new resistant stem cells are being created and the overall rate of resistant cell creation by the division of sensitive stem cell is given by $\alpha b S(t)$. As before, the already existing resistant cells are growing at rate $\lambda R(t)$. As in Equation 5.2, the overall growth rate of the number of resistant cells is given by the sum of the two terms,

$$\frac{dR}{dt} = \lambda R(t) + \alpha b S(t). \tag{6.1}$$

Coupled with this equation, we have the same equation as before for the growth of the sensitive cells,

$$\frac{dS}{dt} = \lambda S(t),$$

where (as in the derivation of Equation 5.4, p. 125), we assume that the value of α is sufficiently small that transitions to resistance do not materially affect the growth of the sensitive stem cells, mathematically $b - d - \alpha b \cong b - d = \lambda$. Otherwise we would replace λ by $\lambda - \alpha b$.

The solution of the equation for $S(t)$ is unchanged from that of Equation 5.4 and we obtain almost the same solution to Equation 6.1 for $R(t)$ as was obtained before (Equation 5.5, p. 125), i.e.

$$R(t) = R_0 e^{\lambda t} + \alpha b t S_0 e^{\lambda t}. \tag{6.2}$$

Comparing Equations 6.2 and 5.5 it would seem that not much has changed; we have just replaced λ by b in part of the equation. To understand what influence having stem cell divisions that result in non-stem cell progeny has on resistance we must look at Equation 6.2 in a different way. To do this consider the proportion of resistant cells:

$$\frac{R(t)}{N(t)} \cong \frac{\alpha b t S_0 e^{\lambda t}}{S_0 e^{\lambda t}} = \alpha b t. \tag{6.3}$$

If the tumour is a pure stem cell tumour, $d = 0$, and $\lambda = b - d = b$;# where d is not zero, it implies that $\lambda < b$ and that the renewal probability $P < 1$. Equation 6.3 states that the fraction of resistant stem cells will be the same in two tumours systems which have identical values of α and b, *at the same elapsed time.* At the same elapsed time from the start of growth, however, the stem cell compartment size will be greatly different for tumours with different renewal probabilities. We will now return to Example 6.1 to illustrate the effect of random cell loss.

Example 6.1 (*cont.*)

Consider the compartment model which has $P = 0.55$ and 1000 stem cells. As calculated, this will occur after about 72 intermitotic periods. The proportion of resistant cells would be the same as observed in a pure stem cell tumour that had undergone 72 intermitotic periods. At this time the pure stem cell tumour would consist of 4.7×10^{21} stem cells, such a tumour would weigh approximately 4.7 billion kilograms.

Given the frequently observed inverse relationship between size and curability it is easy to see that the result of making a small stem cell compartment take on some of the characteristics of a tumour weighing 4.7 billion kilograms is not going to have a good effect! However, a higher theoretical proportion of resistant stem cells in a small stem cell compartment may still not be many cells, if any. How do these effects balance those already discussed (see discussion prior to Example 6.1), which will tend to reduce the likelihood of resistance in tumour systems that are not totally composed of stem cells?

There is no simple mathematical answer to this since one can construct compartment models of tumour systems that have reduced or elevated levels of resistance compared with pure stem cell systems at the same overall tumour size. This is because the proportion of stem cells in a tumour is dependent on the behaviour of the transitional and end cells and not just on the stem cells. However, we can place reasonable limits on what can be expected to occur in clinical systems. Analysis of epidemiological data for the effect of known carcinogens such as ionizing radiation shows that after exposure to a point source excess cancer is not seen before a latent period has passed. A lower bound for this latent period, assuming the carcinogen immediately produces a single malignant stem cell, is the time needed for a tumour cell to grow to a detectable size, assumed to be about 10^9 cells. Observed latent periods vary with age at exposure and tumour type but are rarely less than 2–3 years in humans. The maximum time to death from cancer after treatment of disease should also provide an estimate of the time required for a very small tumour to grow to a diagnosable size. This maximum shows considerable variability for different tumours; however, the survival curve for many tumour types shows a breakpoint at about 3 years. The breakpoint is a point at which the slope of the survival curves changes considerably. Observation in experimental systems has shown that this seems to occur when the number of surviving cells is small allowing for stochastic variability in growth rates and subsequent time to recurrence. Hence we may reasonably estimate a period of about

3 years for many types of cancer to grow from a single cell to one of 10^9 cells, with the caveat that many take considerably longer. Estimates of the cell division time of human tumours has typically yielded mean values in the range 1–3 days. If we assume an average of about 2 days then that would imply that prior to diagnosis the average tumour has undergone approximately 550 divisions ($3 \times 365 \div 2$). A pure stem cell tumour with $P = 1$ undergoing 550 divisions would contain about 4×10^{165} cells. This number of cells would be sufficient to fill the galaxy with tumour. If the tumour consists of 10^9 cells at diagnosis then each cell in a pure stem cell model would have a 'history' of about 30 divisions. Therefore, each stem cell in a clinical tumour will have about 20 (550/30) times as many divisions in its history as a pure stem cell tumour and t in Equation 6.2 would be 20 times its value for a pure stem cell tumour and thus there would be 20 times the population of resistant stem cells. Under these circumstances, a clinical tumour in which more than 1 in 20 cells were stem cells would have more resistant stem cells than a pure stem cell tumour of the same total size, while one with a lower proportion of stem cells would have less.

Now showing that there are more or less resistant cells in a compartment model of growth does not tell the whole story. As discussed before, resistant stem cells have individually the capacity to become extinct. Therefore, merely having more of them around does not necessarily imply that the likelihood of resistance causing treatment failure has increased. For example, a single resistant cell is sufficient to lead to relapse with certainty in a pure stem cell model whereas 10 resistant stem cells will have a less than 50% probability of causing relapse if the renewal probability is less than 0.517. It is possible to calculate the 'probability of cure' using a compartment model of growth. The 'probability of cure' is now not simply the probability that there are any resistant stem cells but rather the probability that any resistant stem cells present will lead to a viable tumour. The theory required to analyse this problem is a branch of probability known as branching processes and has been applied to diverse problems such as the extinction of family surnames. Unfortunately, the derivation of the appropriate results require a level of mathematical analysis that is inappropriate here; so that we will only quote the relevant result.

If we assume that the kinetic and resistance parameters remain fixed throughout the growth of the tumour, then the calculation leads to a very simple result: the probability of cure, P_C, is given by

$$P_C = e^{-\alpha(N-1)}, \tag{6.4}$$

where α is as before. It is assumed that the tumour begins from a single sensitive stem cell and N is now the number of stem cells and not, as before, the total number of cells. Comparison with Equation 5.20 (p. 134) shows that the compartment model of growth leads to the same equation for the probability of cure as that derived for the pure stem cell model except that we replace the total tumour size by the size of the stem cell compartment.

It is important to note that the amplification of the number of resistant cells is caused by only one characteristic of the compartment model of growth. That characteristic is that cells are 'lost' from the stem cell compartment by their conversion into transitional cells. Any nonselective process of cell loss from the stem cell compartment will result in the same effect when we examine the number of resistant stem cells as a function of the overall number of stem cells in the primary tumour. Therefore, stem cells that die because of insufficient nutrition or are shed into the blood stream will have the same effect as differentiation when we analyse the number of resistant cells in the stem cell compartment of the primary tumour.

The formulae presented were derived using the assumption that the growth characteristics of the tumour remains fixed in time. Observation from clinical cancers in the observable range suggests that their growth rate declines with increasing size, a factor that is often attributed to physical or nutritional constraints on the tumour. Since tumour cells, in particular, have limited capacity to alter their mitotic interval, it seems reasonable to conclude that the reduction in growth rate is associated with increased 'loss' from the stem cell compartment. Treating such tumours has the effect of reducing the size and overall nutritional need of the remaining tumour cells so that remaining resistant cells are presumably left in an environment in which cell loss is less than that in the environment in which they previously existed. This, of course, would have a negative effect on the calculated probability of cure, since under the worst possible case the slowing down of the growth rate may be the result of increased cell loss, which is then associated with a greater number of resistant cells; these then persist after treatment since they are now in an environment where cell loss is much less. In this situation Equation 6.4 will overestimate the probability of cure.

The effect of cell loss on the acquisition of resistance is one of the few quantitative phenomena that is not shared by the random mutation and directed mutation models. The directed model of resistance just depends on the number of cells present and not upon their history of divisions, so that under this model the number of resistant cells will be independent of the number of divisions prior to drug exposure. However, this difference is not easily exploited to distinguish between the models for two reasons. Firstly, one would require an experimental model in which it was possible to produce significant amounts of cell loss without changing α. Secondly, most measurements of resistance utilize the survival of clones, which is dependent on (what we have called) the cure probability, a quantity that is unaffected by constant levels of random cell loss.

6.3   Absolute resistance

In the preceding chapter we discussed resistance as if it were an absolute phenomenon, whereas as noted in other chapters resistance to most drugs is a relative phenomenon. For most drugs, 'sensitive' or wild-type cells appear to obey the log kill law. Each cell has a probability of surviving administration of the drug and that probability is inversely related to dose. In most cases 'resistant' cells seem to obey the same law except that a higher dose of drug is required to produce the same probability of cell kill. Indeed in most experimentally studied cases there are no single sensitive and resistant states but a spectrum exists in which cells display ranging sensitivity to drug therapy. The application of drug divides this spectrum into two parts labelled sensitive and resistant, which are determined by the cell type, drug and concentration of use. By the stepwise exposure of surviving cells to increasing doses of drug, cell lines can frequently be created that are resistant to almost any level of drug. In clinical cancer, resistance does not need to be of high order but must be of sufficient magnitude that cells are able to maintain their numbers in the presence of therapy. Since therapy must be scheduled to permit other normal tissue systems to continue to maintain themselves, it is only necessary that resistance among tumour cells be of the same magnitude as the most sensitive of the host's normal tissue systems. Therefore, resistant cells are only required to 'regress' to the normal level of resistance displayed by host tissue to such drugs in order to survive.

Mathematically it is possible to model the effect of less than absolute resistance in the same way as for sensitive cells in terms of the effect of drug therapy on pre-existing cells. The mathematics is beyond the scope of this book but has been explored by several authors. A more tricky problem is how you model the development of the resistance spectrum. This has been undertaken by relatively few authors and has been done in cases where it is possible to identify some discrete change (e.g. gene amplification) that can be associated with the inherent degree of resistance. Essentially it is assumed that the cell may exist in one of a larger number of discrete states that may be ordered in terms of their inherent level of resistance. Then cells are assumed to move between these states in the same way as we have described for the two-state (sensitive–resistant) model, i.e. with a finite probability at each division. Analysis of experimental data has indicated that the values of α associated with transitions between adjacent levels of resistance seem to increase as the degree of resistance increases. Thus high levels of resistance may be achieved at a much higher rate than might otherwise be expected. However, because of mathematical parallels between this phenomenon and that of MDR we will defer further discussion of this topic to that section.

6.4   Uniform growth of cells

We have assumed that resistant and sensitive cells grow uniformly and identically so that their only difference is their susceptibility to drug-induced death. However, alterations that confer drug resistance may be expected to affect other parameters of cell behaviour. Cell growth rate is one such easily measured parameter and doubling times of resistant cells to different drugs have been measured and found to differ from the parental line: usually they are greater but occasionally less. Other things being equal, one would expect, *a priori*, that parental cells would have faster growth rates than variant cells (where we are interested in variants that are resistant) since the population would eventually be dominated by cells that divide fastest. Such ecological considerations are likely to apply to tumour lines that are repeatedly passaged or otherwise maintained since cells with even a small growth advantage then have time to become the dominant type. Therefore, it is no surprise that observation in experimental tumours has more often found that resistant (especially very resistant) cells grow slower than a parental sensitive tumour line. Since faster growth can also be an effective form of resistance to low levels of drug, we may expect some resistant cells to display increased rates of growth. When dealing with clinical cancer, each patient has a unique tumour, and wide variation in the growth rates of individual cancers is observed. We, therefore, cannot *a priori* conclude that resistant cells will necessarily grow faster, slower or even the same as the parent line.

What is the effect of differential growth rates? They can have a number of effects. Under the random mutation model, early creation of resistant cells leads to much greater total numbers of resistant cells than would be the case if they occurred later. The 'magnification' produced by subsequent growth was shown to be the factor that made the random and direct cell models distinguishable by the fluctuation test. Obviously slower growth rates for resistant cells reduces the level of magnification and make the two models more difficult to distinguish by the test. Conversely, more rapid growth rates of resistant cells will cause greater magnification. Increased variability between identical experiments is a consequence of the random mutation model, and such variability will be increased by more rapid growth of resistant variants. An obvious consequence of altered growth kinetics of resistant cells is that tumours which recur after treatment will be kinetically different from the tumour prior to treatment (Section 8.5).

6.5 Variability between tumours

Two of the main qualities sought in an experimental tumour system are stability and consistency of its properties. Clearly such a system must mimic the behaviour of human cancer to a large degree, but an unstable system does not represent a suitable experimental platform from which to explore phenomena. Human cancer goes through no such selection process. Each cancer must have some minimal properties in order to make it 'cancer like' but there is no requirement that the group of human lung cancer should be as consistent in its properties as, for example, the Lewis lung carcinoma animal model. What does this inhomogeneity imply? At a very naive level it could be used to explain every property of clinical cancer: Mr X's tumour is resistant and has metastasized to the liver because Mr X's tumour is just like that. This explanation has no scientific merit and does not assist us in understanding what are the causes of heterogeneity of response.

A first step can be taken by considering how we might generalize the resistance selection model to accommodate heterogeneity. The most obvious way is to require the process to be as before but to permit the parameters involved to differ among tumours. The two central parameters we have recognized so far, which determine the level of resistance, are the size of the tumour N (or more precisely the number of stem cells) and the likelihood of spontaneous resistance α.

When a patient presents with cancer it is frequently difficult to determine precisely their total burden of cancer cells. Although the influence of total tumour burden on the likelihood of resistance is strong, it operates more on a logarithmic than a linear scale so that an estimate that is within $\pm 20\%$ provides an acceptable estimate even though this may represent uncertainty of the order of billions of cells. In some cancers, such as those of the lung, it is feasible to measure the tumour burden within this tolerance so it is possible to standardize these tumous by size. Even in such cases it is not possible, with any accuracy, to identify what proportion of a tumour's size is composed of stem cells so the stem cell burden can be estimated with little accuracy. In many treatment situations, indeed many of those in which chemotherapy results in significant numbers of cures, the tumour burden can only be guessed. A significant example of this is the adjuvant therapy of breast cancer, where chemotherapy is given to treat micrometastatic tumour deposits that cannot be detected but which are suspected to be present because of the experience of other patients with the same cancer. In such cases, treatment is applied to a heterogeneous group. Some will have no cancer cells and, therefore, not benefit from this extra adjuvant therapy. Some will have large numbers of cancer cells, many of which are resistant, and, therefore, they will receive no permanent benefit from chemotherapy. The therapy will benefit those persons with tumours containing no resistant cells that can be eliminated before growing sufficiently to develop resistance and become unamenable to treatment. The preceding gives a flavour of how heterogeneity in tumour size may influence curability, but are such effects quantitatively important? Experimental evidence (Section 5.5) unambiguously indicates the importance of tumour size; however, few detailed calculations have been performed. The following example gives one of them and shows how strong the effect of heterogeneity can be.

6.6   An example from breast cancer

Breast cancer is a tumour in which chemotherapy has been shown to offer significant long-term survival advantages. Individuals presenting with disease that has spread to the lymph nodes, but with no evidence of spread to more distant sites, benefit from the application of chemotherapy after the primary tumour is removed. Experience with breast cancer, prior to the routine use of chemotherapy, showed that some women had recurrent disease soon after surgical removal of the primary tumour in the breast whereas others were disease free for several years before they too recurred. Although some of this variation may be attributed to differing growth rates of residual tumour between individuals, much must be attributed to varying levels of postsurgical tumour burden. Those with more disease recur first, and those with little disease after surgery recur last, if at all. The origins of this variation represent an interesting area of cancer biology and will not be pursued here; what will be developed is the influence of such variation on the affect of treatment. Such variation in size will obviously affect the potential that any woman will have resistant cells present and that their tumour can be cured by chemotherapy. Now we undertake a quantitative estimate of this problem using published data.

Table 6.1 provides estimates of postsurgical tumour burden by menopausal status and number of positive lymph nodes for a group of women treated for breast cancer by surgery alone. These estimates were calculated by Howard Skipper using data on the time to recurrence of these women (Skipper, 1979). He assumed that within each menopausal group the rate of regrowth was uniform. Since this is unlikely to be true, the estimates probably indicate greater variability in postsurgical tumour burden than there actually is, because all variability in time to recurrence is ascribed to differences in tumour burden. However, it is obvious that the variation in postsurgical tumour burden is huge. The prognostic groups (number of nodes, menopausal status) do have differing estimates of postsurgical tumour burden indicating their potential value in separating breast cancer patients into more homogeneous subgroups. However, the prognostic factors used in the table do not succeed in grouping subjects into homogenous groups in terms of residual tumour burden. For example, equal numbers of postmenopausal women in this series with four or more positive nodes are estimated

Table 6.1. *Estimated distribution of postsurgical tumour burden for 716 women diagnosed and undergoing mastectomy for breast cancer, by menopausal status and number of positive lymph nodes*

Tumour burden	Premenopausal No. positive nodes			Postmenopausal No. positive nodes		
	0	1–3	≥ 4	0	1–3	≥ 4
0	0.69	0.31	0.12	0.74	0.35	0.15
$1–10^1$	0.07	0.22	0.11	0.05	0.10	0.08
$10^1–10^2$	0.00	0.07	0.03	0.01	0.03	0.04
$10^2–10^3$	0.04	0.02	0.03	0.02	0.00	0.03
$10^3–10^4$	0.03	0.04	0.09	0.02	0.08	0.04
$10^4–10^5$	0.01	0.07	0.14	0.02	0.06	0.05
$10^5–10^6$	0.04	0.07	0.13	0.03	0.08	0.08
$10^6–10^7$	0.08	0.09	0.07	0.04	0.09	0.20
$10^7–10^8$	0.03	0.11	0.18	0.03	0.11	0.20
$\geq 10^8$	0.00	0.01	0.11	0.04	0.08	0.14
Total	1.00	1.00	1.00	1.00	1.00	1.00

to have no residual tumour cells and to have more than 10^8 residual tumour cells.

Referring to our basic relationship, the probability of cure (Equation 6.4) is given by

$$P_C \cong e^{-\alpha(N-1)} \cong e^{-\alpha N},$$

assuming that all sensitive cells can be eliminated. Using this formula directly is not strictly valid, and we should calculate the probability that a randomly chosen piece of residual tumour containing N(stem) cells will not contain any resistant cells. The formula used is the probability that any *de novo* tumour of N(stem) cells will contain no resistant cells. The difference is small and so we will ignore it. The equation suggests that most (stem cell) tumour burdens of N less than $0.1 \div \alpha$ will be cured by chemotherapy (since $P_C = e^{-\alpha(0.1/\alpha)} = e^{-0.1} \cong 0.90$) and that most greater than $3 \div \alpha$ will not (since $P_C = e^{-\alpha(3/\alpha)} = e^{-3} \cong 0.05$). Substituting $0.1 \div \alpha$ into the formula for P_C and substituting $3 \div \alpha$ yields $P_c = 0.90$ and $P_c = 0.05$, respectively. If we make the oversimplification that if $N > \alpha^{-1}$ the tumour is incurable and if $N < \alpha^{-1}$ the tumour is curable, then we would predict that women with a postsurgical tumour burden $< \alpha^{-1}$ would have their disease cured by a combined regimen of surgery and adjuvant chemotherapy. Here α^{-1} is the average size of the tumour at which it becomes incurable. This is equivalent to assuming that a tumour is always curable prior to the average and always incurable after. All those with no postsurgical tumour burden are cured by surgery alone regardless of the use of chemotherapy.

As an example, if we have a drug that has a value of α of 1×10^{-5} for tumours of women with breast cancer then reference to Table 6.1 would suggest that somewhere around a further 15% of premenopausal women with no nodes involved can be cured by use of the drug (since it is estimated that 15% of such breast cancers have a tumour burden less than $10^5 (= (1 \times 10^{-5})^{-1} = \alpha^{-1})$ but greater than zero) whereas that figure would be about 40% for premenopausal women with four or more positive nodes. The pattern of these estimates are in agreement with what is seen in the treatment of breast cancer; that is, individuals with more positive nodes benefit more from adjuvant therapy. This pattern exists because the distribution of the amount of residual disease is similar amongst the groups for people who do have residual disease. However the likelihood of having postsurgical disease present varies greatly between the groups. Therefore, the different pattern, or variation, in the disease distribution between these groups predicts quite different magnitudes of clinical effect, in accord with a pattern that is observed.

The preceding analysis is not very surprising. It emphasizes the critical role played by the magnitude of disease. Heterogeneity in residual tumour is expected to create heterogeneity in outcome. However, heterogeneity can have more subtle effects, as will now be explored using a calculation based upon the data presented. This will consider the effect of advancing the time of initiation of chemotherapy.

Since the size of the tumour is a critical determinant of chemotherapy success and the tumour grows, we can infer that giving chemotherapy earlier, other things being equal, should improve the outcome. This relationship is clear when resistance is the primary reason for chemotherapy failure, since from Equation 6.4 we have

$$P_{\mathrm{C}} = \mathrm{e}^{-\alpha(N-1)} \cong \mathrm{e}^{-\alpha N},$$

so earlier administration reduces N and increases P_{C}. If we ignore temporarily heterogeneity in N and assume that all systemic treatment failures arise because of drug resistance then we may estimate the quantity αN by inverting Equation 6.4 and substituting observed cure rates, i.e.

$$\alpha N = - \ln \text{ (observed cure rate)}. \tag{6.5}$$

Having an estimate of αN we could use this to estimate either α or N if we knew the other quantity. This is more than we need at present and we will content ourselves with an estimate of αN.

In subsequent studies of premenopausal node-negative breast cancer in the same population it was found that the addition of chemotherapy increased the 5-year survival rate to 84%. If we make the simplifying assumption that the 5-year disease-free rate equals the cure rate (the same assumption that was made in the analysis of residual tumour burdens) then we may estimate the cure rate associated with the addition of chemotherapy. We know that 69% are cured by surgery alone (since they have no residual disease, see Table 6.1) so we estimate that chemotherapy cures 48% ($= [84 - 69] \div [100 - 69]$ of the remainder. Utilizing Equation 6.5 we have

$$\alpha N = - \ln(0.48) = 0.73.$$

Table 6.1 indicates that there is a wide variation in the postsurgical tumour burden; however, for the moment let us consider it to be the same for everyone not cured by surgery alone, i.e. the 69% not cured by surgery have uniform postsurgical tumour burden, N. Now, N in the above equation is not quite the postsurgical tumour burden but the burden present at the time of the initiation of chemotherapy, which is some time after the surgery. By advancing the time of treatment we have a method for effectively shrinking the size N in this formula. Of course this is not real shrinkage; we are just treating the tumour earlier when it is smaller. We can even apply the chemotherapy before surgery, and even though the total tumour is bigger then, the portion of it that will not subsequently be removed by surgery is smaller. Implicit in this reasoning is that the tumour cells which the chemotherapy is required to eliminate are those widely disseminated cells that will not be affected by the primary surgery. At this juncture, the tumour doubling time is not known, but we estimate that we may be able to advance the time of chemotherapy by 30 days, which should result in one less tumour doubling and perhaps as many as three. Accordingly, the size at earlier treatment, N^*, will be in the range $N \div 8$ to $N \div 2$. Therefore, the product αN^* will be in the range

$$0.09 \cong 0.73/8 \leq \alpha N^* \leq 0.73/2 = 0.37.$$

We can substitute these values into the probability of cure equation to obtain estimates of the range of potential cure rates if the chemotherapy is given 30 days earlier. Performing this substitution yields

$$0.91 = e^{0.09} \geq P_C = e^{-\alpha N^*} \geq e^{0.37} = 0.69.$$

These cures only occur among the group (31%) not cured by surgery alone, and the overall rate of cure for surgery plus chemotherapy is given by $0.69 + 0.31 \times P_C$. We predict that the overall cure rate would be in this range

$$0.97 = 0.69 + 0.31 \times 0.91 \geq \text{overall rate of cure}$$
$$\geq 0.69 + 0.31 \times 0.69 = 0.90.$$

Therefore, by giving the chemotherapy earlier we anticipate an increase in the long-term survival rates of at least 6% (90 − 84%) and perhaps as much as 13% (97 − 84%). These are very significant improvements for modest alterations in the way treatment is given! However, these estimates assumed that the postsurgical tumour burden was uniform in those not cured by surgery. If variability in tumour burden is small, then one would anticipate that the results of the analysis based upon a fixed tumour size will still hold. Conversely, if variability is great then the individual postsurgical burden will be the prime determinant of chemotherapy outcome. A precise estimate of the effect of the estimated heterogeneity in tumour burden requires a fair amount of mathematics; however, we may get an approximate answer using the following reasoning.

As earlier in our discussion, we assume that for $N < \alpha^{-1}$ the tumour is curable; this is equivalent to saying that for $\alpha N < 1$ the tumour is curable. Similarly, assume the tumour is incurable for $\alpha N > 1$. Observing a cure rate of 84% one would then infer that the 84% of individuals with the lowest tumour burdens would be those cured while the remaining 16% with greater burdens would not. Using the appropriate column of Table 6.1 we find that women with tumour burdens less than or equal to 10^5 constitute 84% of the women with premenopausal node-negative breast cancer. If we now advance the time of first chemotherapy by 30 days to premenopausal women with node-negative breast cancer then this change does not alter the outcome in the 84% of women with tumour sizes less than 10^5 cells. Similarly it does not alter the outcome in the 11%

with tumour sizes of more than 10^6 cells since even at the most an eight-fold reduction (achieved by earlier treatment) will not reduce a tumour of 10^6 cells below the threshold of 10^5 cells that will make it curable. If we further assume that the distribution of the sizes of the individual tumours in the 10^5–10^6 range are uniform on a logarithmic scale (i.e. there are as many in the range 1×10^5 to 2×10^5, as 2×10^5 to 4×10^5, as 4×10^5 to 8×10^5, etc.) then about 3% of the total (80% of the 4%) would be reduced below the 10^5 threshold by an eightfold reduction and 1% (20% of the 4%) by a twofold reduction. We would, therefore, predict that there would be an increase in the long-term survival rate of 1–3% in the total group achieved by advancing the time of chemother-apy. We can see that these estimates are much below the 13% and 6% predicted when heterogeneity in tumour burden is ignored. Perhaps most importantly, an increase of 13% is in the range where current clinical trials can be expected to detect it, and 3% (maximum!) is not. Trials that have attempted to assess the effect of the early application of chemotherapy in breast cancer (so-called neo-adjuvant chemotherapy) have generally not shown any positive benefit. The preceding analysis seems to indicate that, from the viewpoint of drug resistance, these results are to be expected.

The above calculation is essentially confirmed by more complex models that attempt to use a more complete description of the post-surgical tumour volume and use the true dependence of P_C upon N rather than a simple cut-off. These calculations emphasize the critical role of the distribution of tumour burden in the group of patients under consideration. For example, consider a theoretical distribution of tumour burden as illustrated in Fig. 6.1. Improving treatment from one that will cure tumours of less than 10^4 cells to one that will cure tumours with less than 10^6 cells will result in a large increase in the observed cure rate because there are many tumours in this size range. Conversely, a further improvement to cure tumours of less than 10^8 cells will result in a modest additional increment in the observed cure rate because of the relative paucity of tumours in the size range that would be affected. The actual improvement in cures is dictated by the 'peaks and valleys' of the size distribution rather than the improve-ments in drug efficacy as measured by the log kill or resistance (α) parameters.

The preceding extended example has shown how including variabil-ity in factors known to determine outcome of treatment in experimental

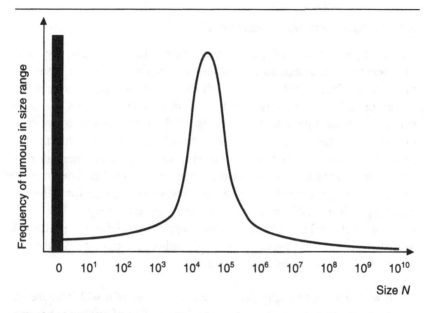

Fig. 6.1 Schematic depicting a hypothetical tumour burden distribution for a solid malignancy after surgical removal of the primary. In a substantial proportion of subjects, all tumour cells are removed at surgery and this proportion is represented by the solid bar at $N = 0$ cells. The rest of the subjects have residual burden indicated by the continuous plot, with a substantial proportion of them having burdens clustered around 10^5 cells. The use of adjuvant chemotherapy is of no value in those with 0 residual burden. The potential value of the chemotherapy to eliminate disease is approximately equal to the proportion of persons who have disease that lies in the range $[1, \alpha^{-1}]$, where α is the transition rate to resistance for the chemotherapy used.

cancers can influence the predicted benefit of changes in therapy. The clinical observation that there is considerable variability in the response to neo-adjuvant treatment of breast cancer does not require invoking a variety of host or tumour factors to explain it. Correct application of the laws derived from experimental cancers are sufficient. Of course this is not to say that all phenomena can be explained but rather to emphasize that naive application of the relationships derived from experimental cancers may be misleading.

6.7   Variability in mutation rates[†]

The other parameter in the probability of cure relationship is α. We have assumed that α is fixed, so that all tumours of the same type have the same value. One could argue that all tissues should have very similar values of α if the property which confers resistance relates to some strongly regulated genetic characteristic. If the characteristic is not biologically important it may vary greatly, both between and within individuals. However, as has been extensively discussed elsewhere in this book, cancer appears to be a disease of genomic instability. The amount of instability is a variable quantity and seems to change for different tissue types. The instability appears to accrue progressively and stochastically so that the level of the instability cannot be definitely predicted from the site, extent or histopathological grade of the tumour. What does this mean in terms of the random mutation?

1. It would seem to imply that the average value of a will increase as the tumour ages, reflecting the cumulative effect of multiple changes in the genome of the tumour cells. Mathematically we would write that $\alpha = \alpha(t)$, the parameter varies with time, and we would expect that if $t_1 > t_2$ then $\alpha(t_1) > \alpha(t_2)$: the rate increases as the tumour grows.
2. It would seem to imply that individual cell lines will develop within the tumour, some with considerable instability while others have less. Accordingly, postulating a single α or $\alpha(t)$, may not be appropriate; it may be more meaningful to consider a family of $\alpha(t)$ parameters, each possessed by one or more cells in the tumour. Although this may be a more realistic model for the development of drug resistance, it can only tell us something if either we specify what this family will be or we can empirically measure it. Neither appears to be possible at this time.
3. It does seem reasonable to assume that different tumours will have different values of α (or families etc.).

We can examine these ideas in a mathematical way as follows. Consider Equation 6.1 for the mean number of resistant cells

---

[†] This section presents some exploratory mathematical material and can be omitted on a first reading.

$$\frac{dR}{dt} = \lambda R(t) + \alpha bS(t).$$

This equation holds even when α varies with time, i.e. $\alpha = \alpha(t)$, so that

$$\frac{dR}{dt} = \lambda R(t) + \alpha(t)bS(t).$$

If $\alpha(t)$ becomes too large it will begin to interfere with the growth of the sensitive cells (i.e. so many sensitive cells will be spontaneously acquiring resistance that the net growth rate of the sensitive cells will diminish). However, if we ignore this then we may continue to write

$$\frac{dS}{dt} = \lambda S(t).$$

As before this yields

$$S(t) = S_0 e^{\lambda t}.$$

Substituting this into Equation 6.1 we obtain

$$\frac{dR}{dt} = \lambda R(t) + \alpha(t)bS_0 e^{\lambda t}. \tag{6.6}$$

We are fortunate in that this equation may be generally solved. The solution is

$$R(t) = R_0 e^{\lambda t} + bS_0 e^{\lambda t} \int_0^t \alpha(u)du. \tag{6.7}$$

The mathematically sophisticated reader will be able to see that the relationships we found previously are a special case of the solution above when $\alpha(t)$ is constant. The integral (du) in Equation 6.7 is equal to the area under the graph of $\alpha(t)$ versus t. The integral has been termed antidifferentiation and provides an alternative way of expressing relationships could also be written in terms of the differential calculus. Integrals also provide estimates of the area under curves that provides a more intuitive idea of their meaning. When α is constant the area under the graph is given by αt, which is the solution found in Equation 6.2. Clearly the behaviour of the solution will depend on what $\alpha(t)$ looks like. The whole point of our development was that $\alpha(t)$ would tend to increase as the tumour grows and contains cell sublines with increasing genetic instability. The most obvious way, at least mathematically, to model this would be to assume that the rate would increase linearly with time, i.e.

$$\alpha(t) = \alpha_0 + \alpha_1 t. \tag{6.8}$$

where α_0 represents the 'original' rate and α_1 its rate of increase ($\alpha_1 > 0$) with time. Now 'reasonable' values for α_1 would seem to be ones for which the effective rate $\alpha(t)$ is not too high at modest tumour burdens; that is, values of t for which the tumour size is in the mid-range. Obviously the actual value of α_1 will depend on the scale of measurement of t (i.e. hours, days, months, etc.). However if we adopt a convention that we will measure the time scale for tumour growth on a scale of 0 to 1, where 0 represents initiation and 1 lethal burden, then a 'small tumour' would represent about $t = 0.5$ on this scale. This would correspond in human cancer to assuming the lethal burden to be 10^{12}–10^{13} cells and that a small tumour would be around 10^6–10^7 cells. This idea of the size of a small tumour was selected by the range at which resistance seems to begin in experimental cancers, indicating that, in such cases, α is in the range 10^{-7}–10^{-6}. Now if we assume that in the small tumour range the value of α is 10^{-7} then we have

$$\alpha(0.5) = \alpha_0 + 0.5\alpha_1 = 10^{-7},$$

so that $0 \leq \alpha_0 \leq 10^{-7}$ and $0 \leq \alpha_1 \leq 2 \times 10^{-7}$. The most extreme pairs of values are $\alpha_0 = 10^{-7}$, $\alpha_1 = 0$ and $\alpha_0 = 0$, $\alpha_1 = 2 \times 10^{-7}$. The first case represents a stable value for α while the second gives its maximum rate of increase under this model. Now we can examine these different scenarios using the general solution of Equation 6.7. If we substitute Equation 6.8 into Equation 6.7 we obtain

$$R(t) = R_0 e^{\lambda t} + bS_0 e^{\lambda t}(\alpha_0 t + \alpha_1 t^2/2).$$

If we assume, as usual, that there were no resistant cells at the start (i.e. $R_0 = 0$) then we have

$$R(t) = bS_0 e^{\lambda t}(\alpha_0 t = \alpha_1 t^2/2). \tag{6.9}$$

If we examine the two extreme values mentioned above, we get from Equation 6.9 for $\alpha_0 = 1 \times 10^{-7}$, $\alpha_1 = 0$

$$R(t) = bS_0 e^{\lambda t}(1 \times 10^{-7})t,$$

and for $\alpha_0 = 0$, $\alpha_1 = 2 \times 10^{-7}$

$$R(t) = bS_0 e^{\lambda t}[(2 \times 10^{-7})t^2/2] = bS_0 e^{\lambda t}(1 \times 10^{-7})t^2.$$

Therefore, for $t = 1$ (remembering this is the value of t which corresponds to a large tumour) both these extreme values give the same answer! Rather than make the values of α equal for the two extreme models at time $t = 0.5$, we could make $R(0.5)$ equal for the two models. This would change the comparisons at $t = 1$ but would not change the qualitative conclusions provided by the comparison. Further examination of this equation also shows that for earlier times in the history of the tumour there will be more resistant cells in the tumour with a constant rate of development of resistance (α). This arises because of the constraint placed, i.e. that at intermediate sizes the rate must be the same. Unstable systems in this framework have lower rates early in the history of the tumour, and this results in fewer resistant cells overall.

Examining the mean number of resistant cells is one approach to determine the effect of changes in α on the evolution of the tumour. An alternative way is to examine the probability of cure function, $P_C(t)$. When there is no cell loss the probability of cure is still given by the probability that no transitions to resistance have occurred. As before (see discussion leading to Equation 5.19, p. 134) this probability is given by $e^{-\mu}$ where μ is the mean number of transitions to resistance. Now the mean value has a more complex form when a depends upon t; it is given by

$$\mu = \int_0^t \alpha(u) b S_0 e^{bu} du,$$

where S_0 is the number of sensitive cells at time $t = 0$. Finally the probability of cure is given by

$$P_C(t) = e^{-\mu} = \exp[-\int_0^t \alpha(u) b S_0 e^{bu} du] \qquad (6.10)$$

Now once again we can substitute in our two extreme cases that we derived from Equation 6.9: for $\alpha_0 = 1 \times 10^{-7}$, $\alpha_1 = 0$

$$P(t) = \exp[-(1 \times 10^{-7}) e^{bt}],$$

and for $\alpha_0 = 0$, $\alpha_1 = 2 \times 10^{-7}$

$$P(t) = \exp\left[-\frac{1}{b}(2 \times 10^{-7})(bt - 1)e^{bt}\right].$$

Although the formulae for the two extreme cases appear quite different they tend to give quite similar answers For example for a tumour size of 10^7 (i.e. $e^{bt} = 10^7$) we obtain for $\alpha_0 = 1 \times 10^{-7}$, $\alpha_1 = 0$,

$$P(t) = \exp[-(1 \times 10^{-7}) 10^7] = e^{-1},$$

and for $\alpha_0 = 0$, $\alpha_1 = 2 \times 10^{-7}$,

$$P(t) = \exp\left[-\frac{1}{b}(2 \times 10^{-7})(bt - 1)e^{bt}\right]$$

$$= \exp\left[\frac{1}{2\ln(10^7)}(2 \times 10^{-7})(\ln(10^7) - 1)10^7\right] = e^{-0.94}.$$

As before, for the mean number of resistant cells, the probability of cure function shows little variation with the two extreme cases. Hence, we would speculate that a linear increase in the parameter α would have little effect on the development of resistance in the tumour.

Can we, therefore, conclude that genetic instability, per se, is unlikely to lead to tumour properties that are substantially different from those of a tumour system with fixed α? The linear assumption may be too conservative as it seems to imply a regular and orderly increase in the rate at which resistance is acquired. A seemingly equally plausible approach would be one in which genetic instability increases geometrically at each division, so that it may be proportional to the overall tumour size. A geometric, or exponential, model for α could be written as

$$\alpha(t) = \alpha_0 + a_1 S(t). \tag{6.11}$$

As before we may run through the two extreme cases: the first where the mutation rate consists of a fixed component only and the second where it consists of a varying component only. This gives the extreme pairs of values as $\alpha_0 = 10^{-7}$, $\alpha_1 = 0$ and $\alpha_0 = 0$, $\alpha_1 = 10^{-14}$, where we have assumed that $\alpha(0.5) = 1 \times 10^7$, that is the measured rate of random mutation would be 10^{-7} in a tumour of 10^7 cells. If we assume that the growth function $S(t)$ is exponential, i.e. $S(t) = S_0 e^{bt}$, then from Equation 6.7 we have

$$R(t) = bS_0 e^{bt} \int_0^t \alpha(u)du = bS_0 e^{bt} \int_0^t (\alpha_0 + \alpha_1 S_0 e^{bu})du$$

$$= bS_0 e^{bt}\left[\alpha_0 t + \frac{\alpha_1}{b} S_0 e^{bt}\right] = \alpha_0 bt S_0 e^{bt} + \alpha_1 [S_0 e^{bt}]^2.$$

Now for $\alpha_0 = 10^{-7}$, $\alpha_1 = 0$ we have the usual relationship

$$R(t) = 1 \times 10^{-7} bt S_0 e^{bt},$$

and for $\alpha_0 = 0$, $\alpha_1 = 10^{-14}$ we have

$$R(t) = 1 \times 10^{-14}[S_0 e^{bt}]^2.$$

We can calculate $R(1)$ (the number of resistant cells in a large tumour), where we assume that a large tumour contains 10^{12} cells (i.e. $N(1) = 10^{12} = S_0 e^{bt}$). Using the above two expressions we obtain for $\alpha_0 = 10^{-7}$, $\alpha_1 = 0$ (since $b = 12\ln(10) = 27.6$)

$$R(t) = 1 \times 10^{-7} \times 12\ln(10) \times 1 \times 10^{12} = 2.76 \times 10^6,$$

and for $\alpha_0 = 0$, $\alpha_1 = 10^{-14}$ we have

$$R(t) = 1 \times 10^{-14} \times [10^{12}]^2 = 10^{10}.$$

Comparing this with earlier calculations using the linear model shows that the assumption of geometric growth (proportional to population size) leads to a massive increase in the number of resistant cells; as a result, any variation in α as the tumour grows can have dramatic effects on the number of resistant cells seen in tumours of clinical dimensions. The final calculation represents a virtual explosion of resistant cells in clinically sized tumours, resulting in a tumour that would be, for practical purposes, totally resistant.

The model that has been presented for variation in mutation rates is not a convincing one since it fails to capture heterogeneity in α among cells, but rather looks at changes over time. Dependence between mutations rates and other characteristics that influence systemic therapy outcome (e.g. metastatic potential) may serve to exacerbate the effect of the development of resistance. For example, if resistance occurs solely in cells destined to metastasize then the overall value of α will provide little indication of the determinants of the success of systemic therapy.

The reader is wise to be cautious about the value of the calculations presented in this section since they represent 'what if' extrapolations. They also represent bounds on what seems reasonable so that the truth is likely to lie somewhere inbetween even if the assumed forms are correct. They do illustrate that simulation of processes known to occur within growing tumours, (instability etc.) can plausibly explain late-stage magnification of the resistance process without having to postulate unreasonably high values of α in the kinds of situation where they have been measured. We will revisit the problem of high levels of primary resistance in Chapter 8.

6.8   Resistance to multiple agents

Cross-resistance is unfortunately not uncommon because single mechanisms for blocking the effect of a drug can often work to impede the effect of others. The various mechanisms have been discussed in Chapter 3. More rarely, drug resistance is produced by pathways that are independent for different drugs. Even more rarely we may get collateral sensitivity where cells resistant to one drug seem to show more sensitivity to the effect of a second drug than is displayed by the wild cells. The question arises as to how we would model multiple levels of resistance. This issue is of importance as most clinical regimens consist of multiple drugs used in ways so that their individual toxicity patterns to normal tissue do not significantly overlap. We will discuss MDR and multilevel (MLR) resistance separately.

6.9   Stepwise resistance to one or more drugs

Initial experimentation with tumour lines showed that it was possible, in many cases, to select lines which displayed resistance to increasing levels of drug. This was achieved in a series of steps, whereby cells were first exposed at a low drug concentration and those which survived were grown and then exposed to a higher level of drug. Similarly it was possible, once cells with a desired level of resistance to a particular drug were created, to expose them to a second drug and repeat this process. In this way cell lines could be created displaying arbitrarily high levels of resistance to multiple drugs. Note that whether we attempt to create resistance to higher levels of one drug or resistance to multiple drugs the experiments are fundamentally the same. In the following discussion we will use terminology relating to MLR but the same development will also apply to selection of higher levels of resistance to a single drug.

A simple way to model this process would be to ignore its multistep nature and treat resistance to several drugs like resistance to one drug. For example, if we have three drugs, T_1, T_2 and T_3 say, with mutation parameters α_1, α_2 and α_3 then we may consider resistance to all of them simultaneously to have parameter $\alpha_1 \times \alpha_2 \times \alpha_3$. Ignoring the multistep nature of the process would be valid if each cell represented a static target for such transformation. The fact that the compartment consisting of singly resistant cells grows at a faster rate than the overall population makes the preceding approach invalid and we will now describe how the process can be modelled mathematically.

To continue this discussion we will restrict our attention to the case of double resistance where there are two drugs to which resistance evolves by separate pathways, that is, resistance to one does not imply resistance to the second. If double resistance arises as a result of two distinct steps (resistance to each drug) then one of them must precede the other (although not always in the same order). We require that one must come first because if two occur simultaneously with appreciable probability then we have the multidrug phenotype, which is the subject of the next section. Once the cell is resistant to one drug then we imagine it spontaneously acquiring resistance to the second in the same way it acquired resistance to the first. Four states can be defined as follows with respect to two drugs (at fixed doses), which we will label drugs 1 and 2:

R_0: resistant to neither drug
R_1: resistant to drug 1 and not to drug 2
R_2: resistant to drug 2 and not to drug 1
R_{12}: resistant to drug 1 and drug 2.

We assume here and throughout that the order in which resistance occurs does not influence the growth state, i.e. $R_{12} = R_{21}$.

Now by our assumptions a cell may only be in the state R_{12} if it was earlier in state R_1 or R_2. If we let $\rightarrow$ represent transitions between states and we have a cell which is in R_{12}, then it, or one or more of its ancestors, made the transitions

$$R_0 \rightarrow R_1 \text{ and } R_1 \rightarrow R_{12}$$

or

$$R_0 \rightarrow R_2 \text{ and } R_2 \rightarrow R_{12}.$$

If we denote the rate at which drug resistance spontaneously occurs in wild cells to drug 1 as α_1 and to drug 2 as α_2 then we may indicate the rate at which these two events occur as

$$R_0 \xrightarrow{\alpha_1} R_1 \text{ and } R_0 \xrightarrow{\alpha_2} R_2.$$

If we assume that acquisition of resistance to drug 1 always occurs at the same rate, regardless of the original state of the cell, then it would also be true that

$$R_1 \xrightarrow{\alpha_2} R_{12} \text{ and } R_2 \xrightarrow{\alpha_1} R_{12}.$$

However, this need not necessarily be true. If we write these rates more generally as $\alpha_{1,12}$ and $\alpha_{2,12}$ we have

$$R_1 \xrightarrow{\alpha_{1,12}} R_{12} \text{ and } R_2 \xrightarrow{\alpha_{2,12}} R_{12}.$$

By considering the problem in this way we may break the case of multiple resistance down into a number of distinct steps for which we have a simple model.

The case for two drugs looks fairly straightforward; however, the number of pathways grows geometrically with the number of drugs so that for three drugs we have

$$R_0 \rightarrow R_1 \rightarrow R_{12} \rightarrow R_{123}$$
$$R_0 \rightarrow R_1 \rightarrow R_{13} \rightarrow R_{123}$$
$$R_0 \rightarrow R_2 \rightarrow R_{12} \rightarrow R_{123}$$
$$R_0 \rightarrow R_2 \rightarrow R_{23} \rightarrow R_{123}$$
$$R_0 \rightarrow R_3 \rightarrow R_{13} \rightarrow R_{123}$$
$$R_0 \rightarrow R_3 \rightarrow R_{23} \rightarrow R_{123}$$

Each arrow in the above schematic has its own rate parameter (α). Such multistate problems are not simple to solve mathematically but it is clear that whatever the mathematical problems associated with the solution of a general multidrug process, it is soon minor in comparison with the problem of having to determine what the parameter values are.

Unfortunately, a full mathematical analysis of even the double resistance process turns out to be a much harder proposition than might at first be thought. We can calculate the expected number of doubly resistant cells, $R_{12}(t)$, at time t for a tumour with an exponentially growing sensitive cell population. The mathematical formula for this takes on quite a simple form when there are no single or double resistant cells present at the beginning ($t = 0$):

$$R_{12}(t) = \left[\frac{\alpha_1 \alpha_{1,12} + \alpha_2 \alpha_{2,12}}{2} \right] (bt)^2 S_0 e^{bt}. \tag{6.12}$$

Now the term in [ ] in Equation 6.12 can be interpreted as the average of the effective α for each pathway (given by multiplying each separate α in that pathway: for $R_0 \rightarrow R_1 \rightarrow R_{12}$ we have the product $\alpha_1 \times \alpha_{1,12}$

and for $R_0 \rightarrow R_2 \rightarrow R_{12}$ it is $\alpha_2 \times \alpha_{2,12}$); the term $S_0 e^{bt}$ is the number of sensitive cells and the remaining term is a power in bt, i.e. $(bt)^2$. Contrast this with the formula for a single level of resistance, where we have from Equation 5.5 (p. 125)

$$R_1(t) = \alpha bt S_0 e^{bt}. \tag{6.13}$$

For the single resistance case we have a very similar structure: the average pathway (which is just α since the pathway consists of a single step), the number of sensitive cells $S_0 e^{bt}$ and a power in bt. Equations 6.12 and 6.13 have a very similar structure, where the power of the bt term is given by the number of steps in the pathway. Using this apparent structure we might predict that for three drugs the bt term would be $(bt)^3$, which is actually the case. Such formulae (which are simply an approximation) are only valid if each α value is small. It is easy to see why the formula for double resistance contains pathway α parameters that are formed by the multiplication of the individual parameters in the pathway since these represent the net effective rates for double resistance; however, one cannot simply use these net rates in the formula for single resistance since the term in bt is incorrect. Each extra step in the pathway raises this power by one: sensitive cells have a term in bt of $(bt)^0$ ($= 1$), the first level of resistance has a term of power $(bt)^1$, the second level a term of power $(bt)^2$, etc. This causes an acceleration of the development of resistance over what might be assumed from the pathway parameter α. The origin of this effect is easy to understand: the doubly resistant cells are derived, initially, from singly resistant cells. The singly resistant populations is growing faster than the sensitive population by a factor proportional to (bt). Similarly the doubly resistant population will grow by a factor proportional to (bt) faster than the singly resistant population so that they will grow by a factor proportional to $(bt)^2$ faster than the sensitive population etc.

We have previously seen that processes, such as cell loss, can magnify the development of resistance to a single drug and these can be expected to have a commensurate effect on double resistance. Based on our previous analysis of the double resistance process as a sequential pair of single resistance processes, we would expect a compounding effect on double resistance. This is exactly what happens, since the enhancing effect of cell loss on resistance is manifest in the linear term in t. The fact that this is a quadratic term in the double resistance formula indicates that this magnification is squared.

Example 6.2

Consider a tumour system in which there are 10^{10} stem cells and interest is in doubly resistant cells for which $\alpha_1 = \alpha_2 = \alpha_{1,12} = \alpha_{2,12} = 10^{-5}$ and $b = 1$. If there is no cell loss (pure stem cell tumour), the age of the tumour, t^*, is given by the solution of $10^{10} = e^{bt^*} = e^{t^*}$ so that $t^* = 10\ln(10)$. The expected number of doubly resistant cells is

$$
\begin{aligned}
R_{12}(t^*) &= \left[\frac{\alpha_1\alpha_{1,12} + \alpha_2\alpha_{2,12}}{2}\right](bt^*)^2 S_0 e^{bt^*} \\
&= \left[\frac{10^{-5} \times 10^{-5} + 10^{-5} \times 10^{-5}}{2}\right] \times (10\ln 10)^2 \times 10^{10} \\
&= (10\ln(10))^2 = (23.02)^2 = 530.2.
\end{aligned}
$$

In the same way as for single resistance, the introduction of cell loss $d > 0$ causes an enrichment of the doubly resistant cells compared with the no cell loss situation $d = 0$. By analogy with the single drug case (Equation 6.2), we would predict that Equation 6.12 would be essentially unchanged except that the size of the sensitive cell compartment would now be given by $S_0 e^{\lambda t}$ rather than $S_0 e^{bt}$ so that

$$
R_{12}(t) = \left[\frac{\alpha_1\alpha_{1,12} + \alpha_2\alpha_{2,12}}{2}\right](bt)^2 S_0 e^{\lambda t}. \tag{6.14}
$$

Consider the case of significant cell loss, where the renewal probability $P = 0.51$. The overall rate of division is $b + d$ and we wish this to remain unchanged when we consider the effect of loss, so we set $b + d = 1$ (since $b = 1$ when there was no loss). A proportion of these, $b/(b + d)$, result in stem cell additions so $P = b/(b + d) = b/1 = b$ and we have $b = 0.51$. From this we have $d = 0.49$ (since $b + d = 1$). We may now calculate the age of the tumour, t^*, when there are 10^{10} stem cells present, i.e.

$$
10^{10} = S(t^*) = S_0 e^{\lambda t^*} = 1 \times e^{(0.5-0.49)t^*} = e^{0.02t^*}.
$$

Solving this equation yields

$$
t^* = 50 \times 10\ln(10) = 1151.3.
$$

Comparison with the value for t^* when there was no cell loss shows that it takes about 50 times as long to accrue the same number of stem cells. If we now substitute these values into Equation 6.14 we obtain

$$R_{12}(t^*) = \left[\frac{10^{-5} \times 10^{-5} + 10^{-5} \times 10^{-5}}{2} \right] \times (0.51 \times 1151.3)^2 \times 10^{10}$$

$$= 344756.$$

Comparison of this number with that for the no cell loss case shows that there is a proportional increase of about 650-fold in the expected number of doubly resistant cells (344756/530).

We can contrast this with the number we may expect if we naively consider resistance to two drugs to follow the same distribution as resistance to a single drug, except with an α value that is the product of the individual values of each drug, i.e. $\alpha_1 \times \alpha_2$, and ignore the presence of cell loss. In that case we would calculate a mere

$$\alpha_1 \alpha_2 (bt^*) S_0 e^{bt^*} = 10^{-5} \times 10^{-5} \times 23.02 \times 10^{10} = 23$$

cells. Conversely there would be 2.3×10^6 singly resistant cells of each type when there is no cell loss. The presence of cell loss at the same rate as before would multiply both these numbers by 25.5.

Example 6.2 shows that naively considering resistance to several drugs to be similar to a single drug will lead to a large underestimation of the number of doubly resistant cells if we just multiply the α values. The calculation of the expected number of doubly resistant cells when there is cell loss shows that there can be unexpectedly large numbers of doubly resistant cells, which can even approach the number of singly resistant cells in a pure stem cell tumour with the same α values. We would conclude from this development that even a model in which the development of resistance to one drug is totally independent of that to another can have large numbers of multiply resistant cells. Fairly modest propensities for cells resistant to one drug to acquire resistance to a second will increase this further and lead to much greater numbers of multiply resistant cell types.

We saw in Chapter 5 that knowing the mean number of resistant cells does not tell us everything about the process. Useful information is also provided by the probability that there are no resistant cells present, a quantity that was termed the probability of cure. We may now expand this idea to consider the likelihood that there are no doubly resistant cells present as the probability of cure when two drugs are in use. (This concept should be distinguished from the probability that a tumour is cured since cure requires that all cells are eliminated not just the doubly resistant ones.) When there is no cell loss, the probability of cure, $P_C(t)$, is

$$P_C(t) = P\{R_{12}(t) = 0\}.$$

Unfortunately this quantity is not simple to calculate and requires some mathematical development. Most authors have concentrated on obtaining relatively simple expressions for this quantity. One, which is similar to the $e^{-\alpha N}$ expression found for a cure from a single drug, is given by

$$P_C(t) = P\{R_{12}(t) = 0\} = e^{-\alpha*N}. \tag{6.15}$$

where

$$\alpha^* = \alpha_1\alpha_{1,12}[-\ln(\alpha_{1,12}) - 1] + \alpha_2\alpha_{2,12}[-\ln(\alpha_{2,12}) - 1].$$

(This formula is an approximation only, for a more accurate formula the reader is referred to Thompson (1989).) The above formula contains the sum of the products of the individual α values in each pathway multiplied by the natural logarithm of the rate of the second step of that pathway. For our previous example where all the rates were assumed to be 10^{-5}, this would correspond to multiplying the pathway rates by the absolute value of $[-\ln(10^{-5}) - 1]$ or 10.5. Thus α^* from Equation 6.15 is 1.05×10^9. Therefore, as far as the probability of cure is concerned, the effect of this being a two-step procedure is to increase about 10-fold the pathway rates obtained by multiplying the α values for each step. We may also include the effect of cell loss, whereupon we can obtain a similar expression to Equation 6.15 with

$$\alpha^* = \alpha_1\alpha_{1,12}\frac{b}{b-d}\left[-\ln\left(\alpha_{1,12}\left(\frac{b-d}{b}\right)\right) - 1\right] + \alpha_2\alpha_{2,12}\frac{b}{b-d}$$
$$\left[-\ln\left(\alpha_{2,12}\left(\frac{b-d}{b}\right)\right) - 1\right] \tag{6.16}$$

Note that probability of cure is no longer $P\{R_{12}(t) = 0\}$ since we must include the probability that doubly resistant cells can spontaneously die out.

Working out a few examples quickly demonstrates that α^* increases as the rate of cell loss does; as a result the effective overall rate for the development of resistance increases. This will be illustrated using Example 6.2.

Example 6.2 (*cont.*)

Suppose we had $P = 0.51$ so that

$$\frac{b}{b-d} = \frac{0.51}{0.51 - 0.49} = 25.5$$

and $\alpha_1 = \alpha_2 = \alpha_{1,12} = \alpha_{2,12} = 10^{-5}$. From Equation 6.16 the pathway rates $\alpha_1\alpha_{1,12}$ and $\alpha_2\alpha_{2,12}$ will be multiplied by $25.5\times$ $[-\ln(10^{-5}(25.5)) - 1] = 368$ giving a value for α^* in Equation 6.15 of 7.36×10^{-8}. This can be compared with the naive calculation of the product of the two rates as 10^{-10}. Furthermore, and perhaps more importantly, it can be compared with the value of α^* when cell loss is absent, i.e. $\alpha^* = 1.05 \times 10^9$. Unlike the single step case where cell loss had no effect on the probability of cure (Equation 6.15), for double, and more steps, it has a marked effect in the direction of making multiple levels of resistance more likely.

At this point we will summarize what we have found:

1. When we consider multiple resistance as a series of stepwise acquisitions of single resistance then the development of resistance to multiple drugs occurs earlier in the life of the tumour than would be indicated by simply multiplying the rates.
2. The compartment of multiply resistant cells increases at a faster rate than the compartment of singly resistant cells, which in turn will increase at faster rate than the sensitive compartment when all the cells divide at the same rate. The phenomenon of random cell loss will enhance this process so that multiple resistance will occur at smaller tumour sizes than in a pure stem cell tumour with the same single drug α values.

3. It is also apparent that if cells already resistant to one drug are more likely to acquire resistance to a second drug (dependence) then the creation of multiply resistant cells will be further accelerated.

It is important to note that the most common method for measuring resistance and estimating α experimentally is based on clonal survival, which is equivalent, in our analysis, to using the cure function, $P_C(t)$; that is, by observing survival fractions and then using Equation 6.6 (N is known) to estimate α. Cell loss does not influence this function for a single-step resistance process and so it will not influence the estimation of α based on such an experiment (after suitable adjustment for the 'plating efficiency'). The acceleration of the development of multidrug resistant cells will, therefore, not be amenable to direct measurement by experiments that measure the acquisition of single drug resistance. It is not inconceivable that combinations of the above circumstances will lead to situations where the number of doubly resistant cell types approaches levels more associated with single resistance. Given the rates postulated in the example, in the subpopulation resistant to one drug in a tumour with no cell loss grown to 10^{10} cells, approximately 1 in 4300 cells ($2.3 \times 10^6/5.3 \times 10^2$) will be doubly resistant whereas in a tumour with high cell loss ($P = 0.51$) the proportion increases to 1 in 170.

As commented earlier in this chapter, the evolution of single drug resistance that involves not one but a number of distinct steps is akin to the situation of MLR. That is, if the cell must go through a series of distinct steps before acquiring resistance to a drug then the process has a similar mathematical structure to that for the acquisition of MLR. Then the conclusions we have made about MLR would apply to the development of multistep single drug resistance, that is, that it would be accelerated by cell loss and this would affect the cure or survival probabilities. This is not the case for single-step resistance. Also if we were considering resistance to two drugs, both requiring multiple steps, then double resistance would be further accelerated. Should each resistance pathway share steps in common then cells resistant to one drug would have a 'headstart' and the corresponding rate, α, would be greater than in sensitive cells.

One of the principal difficulties in the clinical use of the preceding MLR models is the need to specify many parameters, which are rarely known for groups and, given intersubject variability, are never known in the case of the individual patient. There has, accordingly, been an attempt to develop rules of thumb that may be used to guide clinical practice. The principles these rules contain are valuable; however, their utility is limited since they only indicate generalities rather than specifics.

6.10   Rules for the clinical use of multiple drugs

Optimization and control theory are methodologies used to determine the optimal way to manipulate inputs to obtain the best possible result. This is achieved by quantifying inputs and indicating within what limits they may be manipulated and by specifying a quantified outcome measure that is to be maximized (in many cases the outcome is to be minimized but this makes no difference). Our natural quantification for outcome is the probability of cure (which must include a penalty reflecting toxicity) and our inputs are dose levels, drugs selected and the timing of their administration. However, this is too large a problem to solve properly, with the main encumbrance being the large amount of information that would be necessary to set up the model.

In the absence of a complete model, various authors have attacked aspects of the problem by modelling part of the process and finding the 'optimum control' (the term given to the combination of inputs that will result in the best outcome) for that part. Here we will focus attention on what has been done in relation to resistance to two drugs. The probability that the tumour is cured has been used as the single outcome that it is desired to maximize. What investigators have done is to assume that drug doses are primarily determined by toxicity to normal tissue and drugs can only be given safely up to a certain level. They have assumed that the log kill (or similar) law applies so that doses less than the maximum dictated by toxicity will be less effective and we can consider the dose level to be fixed at this maximum. They further assume that the minimum patient recovery interval specified in the protocol is determined by the dose. Since intervals between treatments longer than the minimum will allow more time for tumour regrowth and the development of resistant cells, any protocol that gives drugs at greater than the minimum intervals will be inferior to one that does not. Accordingly, drugs are given at fixed times determined by the timing and dose of the preceding treatment. It is assumed that both drugs may not be given simultaneously, for if they can it will always be better to give them together (given the other limitations imposed). Although these models do not explicitly require that a specific number of drugs be available, they are illustrated using two drugs and so we will continue that here. The final limitation placed on them is that they assume that one must apply a fixed number of treatments. This is not really a limitation but is incorporated because within this structure the best protocol which gives $N + 1$ cycles of treatment will always be better than the best which gives N etc. This is because we have no penalty for adding excessive treatment so we decide in advance that we will not consider excessive amounts of therapy.

This rather long list of assumptions may be summarized mathematically.

1. We have two drugs, 1 and 2, which are given at fixed doses.
2. Drugs 1 and 2 may not be given together.
3. After each drug treatment is given we must wait a fixed time (depending on treatment given) after which we give another treatment: at that time we may choose to give either 1 or 2.
4. The total number of times treatment is given is fixed.
5. We wish to pick the sequence of treatments (e.g. 122122 etc.) that maximizes the probability that the tumour is eradicated.

This is a limited and circumscribed problem and indeed it is not difficult to find its solution if the relevant parameters are known. However, knowledge of all parameters is seldom known so that one is interested in determining the pattern and underlying structure of the sequence that maximizes the probability of cure, if one exists. Initially, we must ask what is the mathematical expression for the probability that the tumour is cured. As we have said each cell is in one of four mutually exclusive categories with respect to the two drugs: sensitive to both drugs, resistant to drug 1 and sensitive to 2, sensitive to 1 and resistant to 2 and resistant to both. If, as before, we let R_0, R_1, R_2 and R_{12} represent these states, respectively, then cure is equivalent to elimination of all cells in each state, i.e. for some time, t', after treatment is complete we require that $R_0(t') = 0, R_1(t') = 0, R_2(t') = 0$ and $R_{12}(t') = 0$. Of course as usual we think of these counts as stochastic quantities so that the probability of cure, $P_C(t')$, is

$$P_C(t') = P\{F_0(t') = 0, R_1(t') = 0, R_2(t') = 0, R_{12}(t') = 0\}.$$

The question becomes how can we mix and balance our treatments 1 and 2, subject to the constraint that we will only give so much of them altogether, to maximize the probability that the tumour is cured? A detailed discussion of how we can perform these calculations and how parameters influence $P_C(t')$ requires a considerable amount of mathematical development. Rather than pursue this we will discuss what conditions must be met for there to exist a sequence of treatments to eliminate the tumour and what the structure of the optimal sequence looks like when these conditions are satisfied.

Firstly, the drugs 1 and 2 must be able to be given so that eventually $R_0(t') = 0$ (i.e. the sensitive cells can be eliminated); if not the drugs can never cure this tumour so the best sequence will still be a failing proposition. Secondly, if some combination of the drugs can kill cells in R_{12} at a sufficient rate to make their net growth rate negative then continuation of this protocol will eventually eliminate all such cells (and presumably all other cells which are, by definition, more sensitive to either drug 1 or drug 2 or both). Under these circumstances, it is not necessary to develop effective first-line treatment since even recurrences can be successfully treated. However, we may still be interested in such cases since the objective then would be to minimize the amount of treatment required to effect the cure. We are interested in the intermediate situation where cure is possible but not inevitable. This, of course, is the case with many situations of clinical interest. The preceding limitations placed on the effectiveness of the drugs against the tumour correspond to the following requirements.

1. Our protocols must be able to eliminate the sensitive cells and thus 'drive' $R_0(t) \rightarrow 0$ (the number of sensitive cells become zero as treatment continues).
2. Our protocols must *not* cause the doubly resistant cells to be eliminated and thus $R_{12}(t)$ to increase (the number of doubly resistant cells can only increase as treatment continues; we are specifically excluding from consideration a drug sequence capable of destroying doubly resistant cells).

The second of these assumptions may seem paradoxical for if these cells only increase and we cannot eliminate them how can we cure the tumour? By their very nature and our assumption about the drugs available, doubly resistant cells can only increase because we have no effective therapy to eliminate them. We can only cure the tumour if there is a significant probability of there being no doubly resistant cells at the beginning of treatment and we can schedule treatments so that this probability does not decrease to zero. By our multistep assumption, doubly resistant cells originate from singly resistant cells so that we can prevent them from arising by controlling the singly resistant cells and we can minimize the likelihood that new doubly resistant cells will arise if we quickly eliminate the singly resistant cells. We must be able to control cells resistant to drug 1 with drug 2 and vice versa. As a result, we have a third requirement.

3. Each of the two drugs must be sufficiently effective against cells resistant to the other drug, to eliminate all such cells after sufficient drug is applied.

Again situations that do not accord with this requirement will inevitably lead to a tumour which is resistant to any protocol that uses drugs 1 and 2 alone.

These three requirements illustrate what the 'best' use of drugs 1 and 2 will involve as the protocol proceeds: (a) reducing the number of sensitive cells, $R_0(t)$ and (b) reducing the number of singly resistant cells, $R_1(t)$ and $R_2(t)$, in such a way that the development of new doubly resistant cells is minimized. The best way to do this depends on the individual parameter values (for α and the log kills of drugs 1 and 2 in the different cell types); however, it is generally true that better strategies tend to 'interleave' the two drugs so that there is not prolonged repetition of one or the other.

In most clinical applications, the parameter values needed to use this model are, at best, imperfectly known. There has, therefore, been interest in developing rules that give general guidance as to what approaches are more likely to be successful. We will discuss two of these rules here: the 'worst drug rule' and the 'alternation rule'.

6.11   Worst drug rule

One of the best known of these rules is the so-called worst drug rule, which basically says that when you have available multiple 'effective' drugs to treat a cancer then you use the most effective one the least (Day, 1987). This counter-intuitive statement deserves further explanation. Consider a situation where two drugs are available for the treatment of a tumour, drug 1 and drug 2. Assume that drug 1 has a higher log kill than drug 2 (in their usually administered doses) and that they both have similar values of α. Let the log kill of drugs 1 and 2 be 3 and 2, respectively, on sensitive cells and the rate α be 10^{-6} for each drug. Assume that the recovery interval after each drug is the same and regrowth between repeat applications of each drug is 0.25 logs. If the tumour is of size 10^{10} cells then four applications of drug 1 (total log kill of 12) will kill all sensitive cells. However, it will require six applications of drug 2 to achieve the same result (12 log kill). Therefore, if we had chosen to give drug 1 six times, the last two applications of it would have been useless because although many cells would exist after the fourth application they would all be resistant. Conversely, if drug 2 were used, there would still have been sensitive cells during the last two applications of it so that its continued use would have been justified. In this way, we achieve all the effect we can achieve with less of the better drug so that we do not need to give as much of it. This is the idea behind the worse drug rule.

It may be countered that the preceding example argues for none of drug 2 because we do not need to give any of it if we have already given four cycles of drug 1. This is correct when we only consider its effect on the sensitive cells, but there are other reasons for using the second drug. One of the main ones is that a second drug may eliminate cells that are resistant to the first drug. If drug 1 is the better drug and can eliminate all the cells resistant to drug 2 in two to three cycles then no more of it need be given *if* sufficient quantity of drug 1 is given to eliminate cells resistant to drug 1 and the remaining cells sensitive to both drugs. Because drug 2 has less kill on cells, generally more of it must be given to eliminate the cells resistant to drug 1 than must be given of drug 1 to eliminate cells resistant to drug 2. Obviously the optimum balance will depend upon the actual log kills and rate parameters.

Empirical tests of the worst drug rule are essentially not possible, since it is more of a guide than a prediction. In order to test it one would want to know all the relevant parameter values (log kills, α values, etc.) to make sure that you had a worse drug. But having done this one would logically not use the rule but go through a detailed calculation and derive a predicted optimum strategy. This strategy would then indicate the best way to use the drugs and the worst drug rule would not be required. The predictions would then be tested to see if they were borne out experimentally. However, this rule is very useful for supporting empirical findings that repeated use of useful drugs will not continue to provide gains in therapeutic value.

6.12   The alternating strategy rule

In contrast to the worst drug rule, which provides an outline of the answer to a general situation, the 'alternating strategy rule' provides a very precise answer to a narrow question.

Very occasionally situations may exist where one has available two drugs that seem absolutely equal in their effectiveness. The question then arises as to how one may optimally use them. This turns out to be a problem to which there is a mathematical solution that does not depend on the actual parameter values. As long as the two drugs have exactly the same values for α and log kill and require the same spacing between consecutive treatments then the optimal approach is to alternate their use (i.e. 121212, etc.). The rationale for this approach is easily understood since we effectively reduce the number of singly resistant cells at equal rates and eliminate them jointly as fast as possible. Also since the two drugs are equally effective giving drug 1 or 2 reduces the sensitive cells by the same proportion so that this compartment is reduced as fast as possible.

Simulations indicate that interleaving early in the protocol has a greater effect than interleaving later in the protocol, so it is more important how a protocol 'starts' than how it ends. The reasons for this is easy to understand. The singly resistant subpopulations are most likely to create doubly resistant cells when these populations reach their maximum size. By interleaving early the singly resistant subpopulations are both controlled and begin to decline. As long as the remaining part of the protocol does not allow either of them to equal or exceed their former size there will be small likelihood that the potential for successful treatment will be considerably diminished.

6.13   Experimental rules

The interleaving strategies contained in the worst drug rule and the alternating rule represent a departure from what has been inferred from studies of experimental tumour systems. Analysis by Skipper and colleagues had suggested the so-called 'treatment to nadir' approach, whereby drug 1 was continually administered until the net-growth rate of the tumour was no longer negative and then drug 2 was repeatedly applied (Skipper, Schabel and Wilcox, 1975). From the viewpoint of the mathematical model, this strategy makes sense: use one drug to eliminate all cells resistant to the other and then switch. However, because the likelihood that double resistance will develop depends on the number of singly resistant cells, it is disadvantageous to eliminate one type while the others continue to grow and it is better to reduce them in tandem using both drugs.

Most experiments that led to the 'treatment to nadir' rule did not include the optimum interleaved strategy so that one cannot really say that there is any disagreement between theory and experimental evidence on this point. Both the worst drug and the alternating strategies indicate that, when resistance is present, considerations based on the behaviour of sensitive cells can be very misleading. The rules indicate that it is the behaviour of the underlying resistant populations which will influence the likelihood of cure.

6.14   Some comments on optimum rules

Mathematicians like optima. And why not, if you can get the best why settle for anything less? However the fact that one strategy, within this context, is optimal and another suboptimal does not imply that there is any practical difference between them. It must be remembered that clinical trials typically only detect differences in cure or survival rates of the order of 0.05 or more. Many strategies may have predicted cure rates within 0.05 of the optimum and therefore be statistically indistinguishable in effect. Also interleaving strategies, per se, are not superior to noninterleaved ones since some interleaved strategies can be very bad indeed. The earlier rules indicate that good strategies will usually involve some amount of interleaving but not the converse.

In clinical situations, patients are unlikely to be homogeneous on those parameters (log kills, α values, etc.) that influence the nature of the optimum therapeutic strategy. It is quite likely that there is no single optimal therapy for the entire population of patients. In such cases, it is possible that the best common treatment strategy, that which produces the best overall result, is not optimal for any of the individuals in the patient population. The obvious approach is to customize treatment to individual patients so that each patient receives the best possible treatment with those drugs available. Unfortunately, there are not any clinical tools that facilitate the measurement of the relevant parameters in a timely fashion. As we have seen, it is treatment given early in the therapeutic regimen that has the greatest influence on outcome in situations where there is a reasonable probability of long-term success. The probability that patients will benefit differentially from the effect of therapy raises the concern that the best overall therapy may not be a suitable rationale for designing clinical protocols. The decision-analysis literature contains several other possible criteria for selecting the best protocols.

In the preceding discussion we have indicated that we wished to maximize the probability of cure and that we would only address combinations of tumour system and treatment where our 'three limitations' held. What happens if we now apply our optimal treatment to systems where cure is unlikely and that the measure of effect will be extension in the survival time? We would hope that the optimal strategies would also perform well in these circumstances too, since the object of both is 'roughly' to reduce the tumour size as much as possible so that either cure is achieved or relapse delayed. The reassuring answer is that optimal strategies for maximizing cure, when it is possible, also maximize the disease-free interval when cure is impossible. Again within the context of this model, the differences in disease-free survival among many strategies in individuals in which cure is impossible is rather small. In fact almost any strategy that utilizes enough of each drug will have about the same effect on the disease-free interval. This observation has two direct implications.

1. In experimental systems disease-free interval is one of the major measures of effect; therefore in evaluating this outcome-measure various strategies will have similar effects (i.e. treatment to nadir and mathematical optima).
2. In clinical studies of patient groups that are mixtures of incurable and potentially curable subjects the differences in effect between optimal and other strategies will be less than in the potentially curable group alone. Potentially curable subjects are those in which the probability of no doubly resistant cells is relatively high at the commencement of therapy (see also Chapter 7).

6.15   Multidrug resistance

The origins of MDR are discussed in Chapter 3 but suffice it to say here that single changes in cell metabolism may confer resistance to the actions of diverse drugs. To the extent that information is known about the origins of such resistance it appears to arise in ways similar to that of single drug resistance. There seems no particular reason to amend the model we presented in Chapter 5 for single drug resistance to cover the case of MDR. All the characteristics developed there merely carry over. As detailed elsewhere in this book, single-step multiagent resistance appears a more common mechanism for resistance in clinical cancer than that which arises in a sequence of steps.

6.16   Summary and conclusions

This chapter has discussed various extensions to the basic random mutation model for drug resistance presented in Chapter 5. By embedding the random mutation model in a compartment model of tumour growth, we have seen how random cell loss acts to age a tumour and make it take on the resistance properties of a tumour of much greater size. This effect is much exaggerated when cell loss is not random and resistance types have growth advantages over parental cells. In extending the random mutation model to multiple drugs we showed that, in cases where such resistance is acquired over a series of steps, multiply resistant types proliferate at an accelerated pace, especially where cell loss occurs, so that even for small values of α, multiply resistant types will be present in tumours of clinical dimensions. The role of genetic instability in furthering the development of resistance was explored and shown to be potent. Inhomogeneity, both between and within individual clinical cancers, was shown to be a primary determinant of outcome.

References

Bush, R.S. and Hill, R.P. (1975). Biologic discussion of augmenting radiation effects and model systems. *Laryngoscope*, 85: 1119–1133.

Day, R.S. (1987). Exploring large tumour model spaces, drawing sturdy conclusions. In *Cancer Modelling*, ed. J.R. Thompson and B.W. Brown, pp. 365–386. Dekker, New York.

Skipper, H.E. (1979). *Repopulation Rates of Breast Cancer Cells after Mastectomy* (Booklet No. 2). Southern Research Institute, Birmingham, AL.

Skipper, H.S., Schabel, F.M. and Wilcox, W.S. (1975). Experimental evaluation of potential anti-cancer agents. XIV Further study of certain basic concepts underlying the chemotherapy of leukemia. *Cancer Chemother. Rep.*, 45: 5–28.

Thompson, J.R. (1989). *Empirical Model Building*, pp. 35–43. Wiley, New York.

Further reading

Buick, R.N. (1984). The cell renewal hierarchy in ovarian cancer. In *Human Tumour Cloning*, ed. S.E. Salmon and J.E. Trent, pp. 3–13.

Coldman, A.J. and Goldie, J.H. (1988). The effects of tumor heterogeneity on the development of resistance to anti-cancer agents and its implication for neo-adjuvant chemotherapy. In *Proc. 2nd Int. Congr. Neo-adjuvant Chemotherapy*, Paris, France, 19–21 February.

Day, R. (1986). Treatment sequencing, asymmetry and uncertainty: new strategies for combining cancer treatments. *Cancer Res.*, 46: 3876–3885.

Goldie, J.H., Coldman, A.J. and Gudauskas, G.A. (1982). Rationale for the use of alternating non-cross resistant chemotherapy. *Cancer Treat. Rep.*, 66: 439–449.

Mackillop, J., Ciampi, A., Till, J.E. *et al.* (1983). A stem cell model of human tumour growth: implications for tumor cell clonogenic assays. *J. Natl. Cancer Inst.*, 70: 9–16.

Mode, C.J. (1971). *Multitype Branching Processes*. American Elsevier, New York. Very mathematical treatment.

Valagussa, P., Bonnadonna, G. and Veronesi, U. (1978). Patterns of relapse and survival in operable breast carcinoma with positive and negative axillary nodes. *Tumori*, 64: 241–258.

7

Clinical predictions of the random mutation model

7.1 Introduction

The random mutation model of drug resistance explored in Chapters 5
and 6 can be used to derive a number of unambiguous predictions about
the behaviour of clinical tumours in response to chemotherapy. These
are basically the same as the ones that were developed from the consideration of the experimental tumours described in Chapter 5 but with
the necessary qualifications. The clinical malignancies are much more
heterogeneous and complex than the experimental systems. One important distinction is that it is not possible to stage clinical tumours with
anything like the accuracy that can be achieved in the laboratory. The
number of actual clonogenic cells in a transplanted tumour can be measured with precision whereas only a very rough approximation can be
made for clinical malignancies. The strongest predictions made by the
model include:

- there will be an unpredictable variation in response to treatment in
  what appears to be identical cases of malignancy
- there will be an inverse relationship between tumour mass and
  likelihood of cure
- combination chemotherapy will be superior to single-agent treatment with respect to the production of cures
- the sequence of drug administration influences outcome.

There are a number of other inferences that can be made from the
model. The above predictions, however, can be considered to be strong
predictions which easily lead from the model and which can be sub-
jected to experimental and clinical tests.

Prediction I There is an unpredictable variation in response to chemotherapy in patients with the same histological type and stage of tumour

The unpredictability of response to chemotherapy is commonly observed in virtually all types of malignancy that are undergoing treatment with chemotherapy. Depending on whether the initial mutations that confer resistance occur early or later in the growth of the tumour, or not at all, a variety of response scenarios are possible. Early mutations will generate a large resistant population and will limit substantially the effect of the treatment. Late mutations leading to a small resistant population will still result in incurability but will probably be associated with complete clinical remission of sustained duration. If no mutations have occurred prior to or during therapy then the tumour population potentially can be destroyed, yielding a clinical cure. All of these scenarios would be consistent with the same average mutation rate to resistance.

Of course, this would not be the only source of variability of response. Constitutional differences among patients in their metabolism of drugs, in normal tissue tolerance to chemotherapy and with regard to any co-existing medical problems may be some of the additional factors that will influence response. Moreover, patients can be said to have identical tumours of histological type and stage only to a degree. Cytological and molecular characterization of tumour types continues at an expanded pace with more and more subtypes being identified. Some subtypes are known to carry a better or worse prognosis than average, and response categories have to be continually subdivided. At the extreme end of reductionism, it is likely that no two cases of human cancer are truly identical. However, with carefully defined groups, the clinical behaviour of tumours is sufficiently similar to make comparisons among individuals feasible and to apply standard treatment protocols to these groups.

Prediction 2 There is an inverse relationship between tumour mass and curability

The function $P(N) = e^{-\alpha(N-1)}$ describes the theoretical change in expectation for cure, $P(N)$, as the tumour population, N, expands. Advanced tumours are less likely to be cured than similar tumours that have minimal clinically detectable tumour burdens. Patients with micrometastatic disease have higher expectations for cure. One sees this relationship across degrees of tumour burden even in very sensitive types of malignancy such as germ cell tumours of the testes. Cancers with large disease burdens of this type (poor prognosis category) have cure rates with standard chemotherapy in the order of 30 to 50%. Medium burden patients have cure rates in excess of 70%, while minimal burden patients (serum marker positive only) are nearly 100% curable. Although it is not possible directly to relate clinical stage of disease to the number of tumour stem cells, in these cases the change from a very high to a low probability of cure in germ cell tumours does seem to occur over an approximately two to three log change in tumour size.

It is apparent that the curability of clinical tumours by chemotherapy quickly falls off as tumour burden increases, even when observation is limited to the clinically detectable range. Change in potential curability with increasing tumour mass does not seem to be a gradually diminishing phenomenon but appears to involve a fairly narrow range of tumour sizes. The most striking examples of this are seen in those tumours where apparent cure is possible in the adjuvant setting (where we are treating a microscopic tumour burden) and where the same tumour is virtually incurable at the time of minimal clinical detection (osteosarcoma, early-stage colorectal cancer, early- versus late-stage breast cancer, neuroblastoma, etc.).

Clinical, radiological and biochemical marker measurements can provide only an approximate estimate of actual tumour burden. It is apparent that even by histological examination the number of tumour cells per cubic centimetre of tissue can vary widely with different types of malignancy. Hodgkin's disease commonly has few identifiable malignant cells (Reed–Sternberg) per histological section, with much of the tumour appearing to consist of reactive and inflammatory cells. In contrast, small non-cleaved cell lymphoma (Burkitt's type) displays sections that are densely packed with small malignant lymphocytes. Compared with Hodgkin's disease, an equivalent volume of Burkitt's tumour might contain one to two logs more actual tumour cells. Even if there were no other differences in the constituent cells, this on its own could account for some of the difference in curability between the two diseases. A further confounding issue with respect to assessing acurately tumour burden in patients is the question of actual number of tumour stem cells present as opposed to simply the number of morphologically abnormal cells.

It will be recalled that in the spontaneous AKR mouse lymphoma there was a great variation in the number of lymphoma colony-forming cells per total malignant cells present (Chapter 2). The range was approximately over three orders of magnitude in different individual mice. Similar ranges in *in vitro* colony-forming efficiency have been seen in human tumour stem cells assays. The relationship between *in vitro* colony-forming efficiency and that *in vivo* is not understood with certainty but a conservative interpretation would be that human tumours must show some variation from patient to patient in the numbers of tumour stem cells per standard volume of tumour.

Despite the difficulties in accurately measuring true tumour burdens clinically, the main lesson seems clear. Potential curability by chemotherapy declines rapidly with tumour size increase and chemotherapy should be initiated at the earliest time feasible and against micrometastatic disease if possible. No other process operating within the cancer cell population appears to mitigate so heavily against successful drug treatment as the progressive increase in cell number with concomitant increase in cellular heterogeneity.

There is a final point that needs to be made regarding tumour size and curability. Small tumour burdens in the sense used here imply a young tumour and not one that has been shrunk down from a larger size. Although the two tumour masses may be the same in these circumstances, the biological age of the two tumours will be quite different. Whatever means have been used to shrink a large tumour will not turn the clock back on its biological age (Chapter 6). If it has been reduced in size by chemotherapy, it can probably be expected to contain a high proportion of resistant cells by virtue of the selection process.

Some kinetic models of chemotherapy would not distinguish between these two states since both tumours would be at the same point in the growth curve function as measured by volume. However, the elapsed biological and chronological time to reach these points would be different, with more cellular divisions involved in the 'shrunken' tumour (the mathematical basis for this is discussed in Chapter 6). The behaviour of the two equally sized tumours would not be expected to be the same and this is abundantly confirmed by experience. (Compare the drug sensitivity of minimal stage Hodgkin's disease with relapsed Hodgkin's that has undergone 'conditioning' chemotherapy prior to bone marrow transplantation.)

Surgical debulking will only change the heterogeneity of the tumour population if most of the tumour cells are present in a few large discrete masses. These masses will presumably be the 'oldest' part of the tumour and probably the most heterogeneous. If these masses are removed by surgery then the residual microscopic disease may contain both a lower proportion and quantitatively fewer drug-resistant cells than were present in the original disease. However, this residual disease will still be potentially more drug-resistant than a 'young' tumour of the same size.

Prediction 3   Combination chemotherapy will be superior to single agent treatment

If we take the function $P(N) = e^{-\alpha(N-1)}$ and replot it with N fixed and varying the value for α, we find that this yields a sigmoid-shaped 'limiting dilution' curve similar to the original function (Fig. 7.1).

For any value of N (the number of tumour cells) the probability of cure diminishes as the mutation rate increases. This is intuitively obvious but what can we infer from this regarding the utilization of chemother-

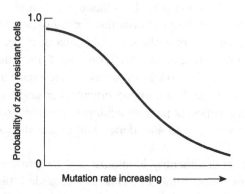

Fig. 7.1. Plot of the function $P(N) = e^{-\alpha(N-1)}$ (this equation should be more properly written as $P(\alpha)$ since P varies with α not N) with N fixed and varying values for α (mutation rate to resistance). As α increases, the probability of zero resistant cells diminishes. Likewise as α is reduced the probability of zero resistant cells (cure) increases. In the limit when $\alpha = 0$, the probability of nonresistance equals 100%. Reducing the value of α can be achieved, in effect, by utilizing combinations of non-cross-resistant drugs, so that the likelihood of any tumour cells expressing resistance to at least one of the drugs is minimized.

apy? There is no apparent way to reduce the spontaneous mutation rate in a biological system other than by applying substances that oppose the action of known mutagens. Unfortunately several of the modalities used in treating cancer are known to increase the general mutation rate in the tumour. The question is to some degree moot, however, as by the time the neoplasm is diagnosed the mutational events of concern will have either occurred or not.

It is possible to deal with this problem without actually changing the spontaneous mutation rate within the cancer. We can, in effect, reduce the probability of there being any drug-resistant cells present by utilizing two or more agents concurrently. The random mutation model provides a strong rationale for the use of combination chemotherapy.

The earliest clinical uses of combination chemotherapy were based on a number of considerations, with the issue of drug resistance not necessarily being foremost. It was felt important to combine together as many drugs that were known to be individually active against the disease as was feasible. Even relatively minor degrees of activity were sometimes felt to be adequate reasons for inclusion in a protocol. Some of the first combination protocols that were found to be useful in certain types of tumour included the so-called 'triple therapy' for testicular cancer (actinomycin D, chlorambucil and methotrexate), VAMP (vincristine, amethopterin (methotrexate) 6-mercaptopurine and prednisone) for acute lymphoblastic leukaemia in children and MOPP (mechlorethamine (nitrogen mustard), oncovin (vincristine), procarbazine and prednisone) for Hodgkin's disease. Early experience with these protocols indicated significant improvement over single agent therapy, with a higher proportion of patients achieving complete remission and a significant proportion, 10 to 40% depending on the disease type, being cured.

Combination chemotherapy is intense and its introduction was not without controversy. A number of clinicians regarded this as mindless, shotgun therapy that was 'an assault against the patient'. There were two common criticisms: if we used a number of drugs simultaneously and there was therapeutic benefit then, 'you wouldn't know which drug had worked'. Another concern expressed was the reluctance to use all known active drugs at the beginning. The treating physician would wish to hold back an agent in reserve to be used as palliation when the initial protocol failed. Of course, withholding a potent agent at the beginning simply increased the likelihood of the initial treatment being unsuccessful.

Considerations that dictated the structure of multiagent protocols included different patterns of toxicity and differing modes of action, including whether drugs acted at different points in the cell cycle. As more came to be appreciated about the presence of drug resistance it was recognized that the use of agents that were not cross-resistant was of great importance. Related to the issue of non-cross-resistance was that of collateral sensitivity, whereby a cell that was resistant to drug A might display increased sensitivity to drug B and vice versa. This is obviously a desirable state of affairs but, unfortunately, seems quite uncommon. Finally, probably in part related to the issue of collateral sensitivity, there is the principle of exploiting drug synergy when it can be identified. True synergistic drug combinations are infrequent but some potent examples have been identified (e.g. cisplatin plus etoposide).

In hindsight, it is apparent that some of the early useful multiagent protocols such as VAMP, MOPP and CMF (cyclophosphamide, methotrexate, 5-FU), incorporated many of these basic principles. Since the time that these first combination protocols were introduced virtually all of the curative programmes of chemotherapy have required multiple agents to achieve their goal. Only a very few types of human cancer appear curable by single agents when treated at an advanced stage (e.g. seminoma, trophoblastic choriocarcinoma and hairy cell leukaemia). Even seminoma and choriocarcinoma yield better results when treated with multiple agents, and the very rare B-cell malignancy hairy cell leukaemia may be a special case with part of the therapeutic effect being mediated by suppression of endogenous B-cell growth factors.

Prediction 4 Certain sequences of drug administration may be superior to others

From the previous considerations, it is apparent that the most effective method of employing cancer chemotherapy is to utilize all of the most active individual agents simultaneously. An alternative approach might be to employ each active agent individually for a set number of courses and then switch to the second, third and fourth agents in order. This would have the advantage of resulting in each drug being given close to its optimum dose. We might then envisage a sequence of 111, 222, 333, 444, etc.

This approach was frequently tried in the early days of chemotherapy and virtually always resulted in treatment failure, even though clinical improvement and some survival prolongation was achieved. From the perspective of drug resistance it is easy to see why this is generally a failing strategy. If we assume that all four drugs are required for cure then we can infer that the tumour at outset will contain at least some cells that are resistant to each of the four drugs individually, e.g. we will have subsets of cells designated R_1, R_2, R_3 and R_4. There could also be cells present that are concurrently resistant to two or three of the drugs, but we will assume that at the outset there are none of these multiple-level resistant cells. A course of therapy with drug 1 will reduce the sensitive cell population significantly and will greatly reduce (or even extinguish) some of the resistant subclones. However, during the period of therapy with drug 1 the subpopulation R_1 will grow unimpeded. It may evolve some doubly resistance cells (e.g. R_{12}, R_{13}) that were not present initially and that will have an extended opportunity to evolve to a higher multiple-level resistant state (R_{1234}) and render the tumour incurable.

If, however, the treatment is applied in 'packages' of all four drugs '1234' then the likelihood of multiple-level resistance will be reduced and this will more than offset the possible reduced log kill produced against the sensitive cells (because of necessary dose reductions when four drugs are used together). Now suppose all four drugs are highly toxic and can be given simultaneously only with very significant dose reductions, to the point where some of the drugs may be being delivered in nontherapeutic doses. It may then transpire that the most agents that can be given together at what is considered to be a therapeutic dose is two, that is 12 and 34. Under the following conditions what is the optimal sequence to employ with the two drug combinations?

1. Drugs 12 and 34 have nearly equivalent log kills on the sensitive cells and on the resistant subpopulations that are sensitive to them
2. The net mutation rate to resistance to produce R_{12} is approximately the same as that for R_{34} and likewise for the sequence R_{12} to R_{123} etc.
3. There exists a degree of non-cross-resistance between 12 and 34. Ideally this should be complete but in practice moderate cross-resistance would still yield an advantage. If 12 was totally cross-resistant with 34 then the effect of alternating them would be equivalent to giving one combination alone (this may be a more common situa-

tion than was originally appreciated owing in part to phenomena such as MDR).

The mathematical considerations given in Chapter 6 show that on average the best strategy will be to alternate courses of 12 and 34 (12, 34, 12, 34, etc.). This will be inferior to giving drugs 1234 simultaneously but if that is not feasible then the one-to-one alternation emerges as the next best solution.

Given these rather stringent requirements it is perhaps not surprising that it has been difficult to demonstrate convincingly that one-to-one alternation constitutes a superior strategy when applied in clinical situations. Of the requirements for the full impact of the strategy to be manifest, quantitative equivalence of therapeutic effect may be the most difficult to achieve. This would basically require testing the two protocols to be alternated against two groups of patients with the same stage and type of tumour. Not only response rates and duration would need to be assessed but also cure. This relates to the fact that the random mutation model makes no strong predictions about the behaviour of the noncured groups, though some inferences can be drawn from the average duration of remission in those patients who ultimately relapse.

Since the protocols have to be assessed for the capacity of cure individually, this implies the desirability of evaluating the strategy in tumour types in which cures with one protocol are possible. Assessment of non-cross-resistance is easier to establish as this simply requires a crossover trial with those patients who display resistance at the commencement of therapy. The very large number of forms of pleiotropic or multidrug resistance, however, make it unlikely that two protocols each containing two to four drugs would ever be found to be completely non-cross-resistant.

It has proved difficult to evaluate rigorously one-to-one alternation strategies at the clinical level. One of the studies that has come closest has been that of Fukuoka et al. (1991) in Japan, who assessed the effectiveness of two sequences of CAV (cyclophosphamide, doxorubicin and vincristine) and EP (etoposide, cisplatin). The study was not ideal as CAV and EP were not separately assessed for their curative potential, though a degree of non-cross-resistance was established. In addition, patients were crossed over to the other arm of the study at the first sign of clinical resistance (an ethical necessity). Despite these problems, the authors were able to demonstrate a small but statistically significant superiority for the one-to-one alternation of CAV and EP compared with a sequence of three courses of CAV followed by three courses of EP.

There have been many tests of so-called alternating chemotherapy, with a few showing moderate beneficial effects but most showing no difference in the treatment arms. Some of the most likely reasons for this have been mentioned. Given the problems of rigorously testing the issue of alternation, it is probable that this particular strategy will remain more of a theoretical approach than a practical solution.

7.2 Optimal design of multiagent protocols

The discovery of a large number of different multidrug-resistant mechanisms poses many difficulties for the design of effective combination chemotherapy regimens. In addition to evaluating agents for their individual activity against a specific type of tumour and for minimizing overlapping patterns of normal tissue toxicity, protocols will need to avoid the use of agents that are likely to be rendered ineffective by the same biochemical alteration in the cell. Previously, it was assumed that if two drugs were different chemically and had differing mechanisms of action cross-resistance would probably not be a problem. The existence of many different multidrug-resistant phenotypes makes optimal drug selection considerably more difficult and also more crucial. If we assume that we have only so much toxicity 'space', then to fill this space with drugs that could in principle be negated by a single genetic change would be highly inefficient. For example, the potent agents vincristine, etoposide, doxorubicin and paclitaxel could all be nullified by a mutation resulting in increased expression of P-glycoprotein (P-gp). It seems likely that increased expression of the multiresistance protein MRP would have a similar effect. It will be important to make use of the available knowledge about the typical mechanisms and patterns of cross-resistance that are seen in specific tumour types. For example, the most common mechanism of resistance to doxorubicin in breast cancer appears to be alterations in topoisomerase II rather than increased expression of P-gp. Under these circumstances, it would be rational to employ paclitaxel in the treatment of doxorubicin-resistant breast cancer or in combination with doxorubicin as primary treatment. Paclitaxel resistance can arise through changes in one of the proteins that make up the mitotic spindle, but this would not affect doxorubicin.

Some of the problems associated with optimal drug selection are illustrated by the results of a large, multicentre study that compared four different combination chemotherapy protocols in the treatment of large cell lymphoma. The standard protocol for the treatment of this malignancy has been the multiagent programme designated CHOP (Table 7.1). In an attempt to improve on the results that were seen with the CHOP protocol (30 to 40% long-term survival) a number of new programmes that combined more intensive dosing with additional numbers of agents were evaluated at single institutions. Three of the most successful of these are indicated in Table 7.1 and, on the basis of the results that were seen in the single institution trials, the decision was made to compare all four protocols in a large, prospectively randomized study.

The preliminary results from the single institutions suggested that it might be possible to improve the long-term survival rate to better than 60% in large cell lymphoma if these more aggressive programmes were employed. However, when the trial was completed and the results analysed, it was found that the new protocols did not yield results that were statistically superior to those obtained with the basic CHOP programme when the latter was used in a consistent standardized manner.

This proved to be a considerable disappointment to many investigators who had felt that the combination of greater dose intensity combined with greater diversity of agents ought to have yielded superior results in what is considered to be a fairly sensitive class of malignancy. Although at this point we cannot be sure of all of the factors that resulted in there being a negative outcome to the study, at least two things immediately spring to mind. It can be noted that all four of the protocols contain at their core the four basic drugs that make up the CHOP program. Two of the protocols, MACOP-B and SC-BACOD in addition contain methotrexate and bleomycin and the most complex protocol, the ProMACE-CytaBOM, contains a further three agents (procarbazine, ara-C and etoposide) that are not contained in any of the other protocols. Leaving aside the issue of peak dose and dose frequency, one might have imagined that the results with the different programmes should have progressively improved as the number of active agents was increased. In theory, the ProMACE-CytaBOM protocol should have yielded the best results with the MACOP-B and SC-BACOD intermediate in activity compared with CHOP.

At the time these protocols were under development, less was known about the problem of MDR and its general ubiquity in many types of

Table 7.1. *Combination chemotherapy for treatment of large cell lymphoma: comparison of the standard CHOP protocol with third-generation protocols*[a]

CHOP	M-BACOD	MACOP-B	Pro-MACE–CytaBOM
Vincristine	Vincristine	Vincristine	Vincristine
Cyclophosphamide	Cyclophosphamide	Cyclophosphamide	Cyclophosphamide
Doxorubicin	Doxorubicin	Doxorubicin	Doxorubicin
Prednisone	Dexamethasone	Prednisone	Prednisone
	Methotrexate	Methotrexate	Methotrexate
	Bleomycin	Bleomycin	Bleomycin
			Procarbazine
			Cytosine arabinoside
			Etoposide

[a] The (considerable) differences in dosage and schedule even for the same drugs are ignored for this comparison. The first four drugs in each protocol are identical (dexamethasone is equivalent to prednisone).

human malignancy. For example, it is now known that etoposide can be blocked by the same mutation that can impede the effectiveness of vincristine and doxorubicin (increased expression of P-gp). Likewise, a mutation in topoisomerase II could neutralize the effect of both etoposide and doxorubicin.

In addition, there have been reports that some multidrug-resistant cells also show a collateral resistance to methotrexate and bleomycin, although this is uncommon. And it is also possible that there is at least a degree of partial cross-resistance between procarbazine and cyclophosphamide. Finally, the drug ara-C probably does not have a great level of clinical activity in the dose schedule that was utilized in the ProMACE-CytaBOM programme.

Therefore, there is a possibility that overlapping patterns of cross-resistance may have largely nullified the impact of the additional drugs contained in the more intensive protocols. The most potent drugs were probably the four components that made up the CHOP program, and these were common to each of the protocols. If the contribution of the other drugs was relatively minor, then the trial may have come down to simply comparing four different versions of CHOP.

Another possibility is that from the point of view of the chemotherapy employed, large cell lymphoma is actually made up of several fairly distinct subgroups. Recent observations suggest that large cell lymphoma, as characterized by molecular studies, is made up of at least two subgroups with one group of T-cell lineage having a very poor response to chemotherapy and another subgroup (B-cell lineage and P-gp negative) being virtually 100% curable. These two subgroups could be considered as being virtually two separate diseases. If one subgroup is highly sensitive to chemotherapy and the other quite resistant, then the proportion of long-term survivors will be dictated by the proportion of patients who fall into the sensitive subgroup. The group that is quite resistant may not be susceptible to chemotherapy of the type and dose that was employed in the more intensive protocols. Under these circumstances, the result would be essentially the same outcome across all four protocols, even though the three third-generation protocols were in a sense 'better'. However, their superiority would only be manifested against a tumour type that showed a spectrum of sensitivity and resistance and did not readily divide into two main subcategories.

There could well be other reasons for the failure of the multiagent protocols to show improved benefit, but the lesson to be learned from this important study is that it is going to be insufficient simply to combine drugs that have individual activity and expect that the consequence will be a superior treatment outcome. More information is going to be needed about the common modes of resistance that are expressed in the tumour population to be treated and, in particular, to identify if there are subgroups that are significantly more or less sensitive to drug treatment than the average.

7.3   The concept of dose intensity

Mention has been made previously of the issue of dose intensity (with respect to the treatment of experimental leukaemia, Chapter 2). In 1984, Hryniuk and Bush published a simple method of calculating the so-called dose intensity of multiagent protocols that would allow comparisons to be made with different protocols and assessments of whether the intensity of applied dosage influenced treatment outcome.

The Hryniuk–Bush algorithm involved taking one of the standard protocols for treating a particular category of malignancy, i.e. CMF for breast cancer, CHOP for large cell lymphoma, etc., and utilizing it as the 'gold standard'. The dosage of each drug in these protocols was arbitrarily given the value of 1 so that the total dose intensity of each would be equal to 3 for CMF and equal to 4 for CHOP, etc. Then the actual doses of the protocol were calculated and normalized to a dosage per body surface area (m^2) per week. The doses were all described on a per week basis even if in the actual clinical protocol the doses were given at two-, three- or four-week intervals. For example, if the dose of cyclophosphamide is given at a level of 1200 mg/m^2 every 4 weeks, then this would be described as equivalent to 300 mg/m^2 weekly. If this particular dose corresponded to the protocol that was the 'gold standard' then a protocol that gave cyclophosphamide at a dose of 600 mg/m^2 every 2 weeks, would be considered to have the same dose intensity (i.e. 1). If the protocol that was being compared gave cyclophosphamide at a dose of 1000 mg/m^2 every 4 weeks then the dose would be considered equivalent to 250 mg/m^2 per week, and the dose intensity of the cyclophosphamide would be 250/300 or 0.83; a protocol that gave cyclophosphamide at a dose of 1600 mg/m^2 every 4 weeks would have a dose intensity of 400/300 or 1.33 (in other words a higher dose intensity than the standard protocol). The *relative* dose intensity for a multidrug regimen is obtained by adding the dose intensities for each drug in the regimen and dividing this by the same quantity for the gold standard.

Using this approach, it was possible to develop dose-intensity scores for a number of multiagent protocols used in clinical treatment. In terms of protocol comparison, it is of most use in comparing protocols that are made up either completely or largely of the same drugs. It would be impossible to do cross-comparisons with protocols that contained different drugs.

In the dose-intensity calculations, we are simply looking to see whether there is an optimal degree of dosing for producing favourable patient outcomes and in particular whether exceeding the standard protocol by still-tolerable increases in dosage is associated with a concomitant improved therapeutic response.

There are, of course, a number of broad assumptions that have to be made in order to carry out the calculation of the relative dose intensity. Firstly, each drug at the dose given in the gold standard is considered to have equivalent effect since proportionate increases in any dose (with reference to the doses in the gold standard) is postulated to have the same effect. Secondly, the dose response curve is linear (e.g. a dose of 2 g once every 4 weeks is equivalent to a dose of 500 mg administered weekly). Both these assumptions seem unlikely to be true in practice, especially when used for different outcomes (e.g. response rates and survival, which are nonlinearly related to one another) so that relative dose intensity is unlikely to be mathematically accurate.

Using this approach, Hryniuk and Levin (1987) were able to demonstrate that there was a good correlation between outcome and administered dose intensity of CMF-type protocols in breast cancer as well as in platinum-containing protocols in ovarian cancer. It was also shown by DeVita and Hubbard (DeVita, Hubbard and Longo, 1987) that there appeared to be a similar correlation between outcome and dose intensity with respect to the treatment of Hodgkin's disease and non-Hodgkin's lymphoma. Other studies that have looked for correlations between dose intensity and outcome in diseases such as small cell lung cancer have not found any.

It must be remembered that virtually all of the protocols that were used in dose-intensity analyses were operating in what was felt to be the therapeutic range for the drugs in the combination. In one study, intentional reduction in dose intensity by a factor of two compared with standard CMF did result in less favourable outcome (Tannock *et al.*, 1988).

At this juncture it appears that dose intensity is a variable that needs to be kept in mind and that intentionally reducing doses to well below the usual standard clinical dosage level will almost certainly have deleterious effects. However, moderate escalations of dose greater than the usual clinical ranges have not been consistently shown to be beneficial.

An analysis by Coppin (1987) indicated that, in addition to dose intensity, there were at least two other variables that probably needed to be controlled in any comparison of protocols. These were the average level of dose given at each treatment interval and, as well, the total amount of drug given as part of the protocol. In other words, the duration of the protocol had to be at least some minimum period of time. In the *reductio ad absurdum* case, a single course of treatment even if it were given with optimal dose intensity would probably fail for the reasons that were noted in the experimental chemotherapy studies of Skipper (1990).

From the point of view of drug resistance, we can also develop the concept of dose intensity but in this case there is one important difference in the conclusions. If preventing the emergence of drug-resistant cells is considered an important objective in treatment (and these have not already emerged at the time therapy has commenced) then it will be the intensity of the first dose and its corresponding log kill on sensitive cells that will be a major determinant of the likelihood of achieving this goal. The dose intensity of later dosages can be reduced or compromised in various ways with much less effect on eventual outcome, but the first dose, which by definition will kill the largest absolute number of sensitive cells, will have the biggest impact on whether the tumour will subsequently develop drug resistance. A formal model for describing the impact of dose intensity on drug resistance is given in Coldman, Coppin and Goldie (1988). In every other respect, though, the dose-intensity equation derived from drug resistance mutations leads to similar conclusions to those found by Hryniuk and Bush (1984) and by Coppin *et al.* (1988).

The importance of dose intensity was initially identified by Skipper, who found that if individual doses were too small or spaced too far apart or if there was an insufficient number of them the result would be treatment failure (Skipper, 1990).

7.4   High-dose chemotherapy

The Hryniuk dose-intensity relationship can be most readily applied when the chemotherapy protocol under consideration consists of a number of treatments given at various time intervals and in which there will be expected periods of tumour regrowth. The special circumstance of a single high-dose chemotherapy treatment followed by marrow stem cell reconstitution does not lend itself to a simple dose-intensity calculation. These high-dose treatments are better regarded simply as dose response effects in which antitumour activity follows the log kill law described in Chapter 1.

It will be recalled that the amount of log kill achieved will depend on the dose of chemotherapy and the value of a parameter which was designated β. This parameter is determined by the killing efficiency of the particular drug (or drug combination) against those cells.

It is apparent from the log kill law that, depending on the degree of relative resistance of the most resistant subpopulation plus the absolute size of that population, massive dose escalation will generate a range of effects from complete cure to negligible cytoreduction. For example, if the standard dose produces a 0.5 log kill then escalation to five times

that dose will produce at most a reduction to 0.003 of the initial population (a 2.5 log kill), which might well be insufficient to eradicate the
resistant subpopulation.

If the relative sensitivity of the resistant cells was such that the standard dose produced a 1.0 log kill then the fivefold dose escalation would
produce a kill more than two orders of magnitude greater than the first
instance (surviving fraction equal to 0.00001). In other words, small
changes in relative resistance will translate into large differences in
cell killing. This underscores the likely futility of attempting to batter a
small highly resistant population 'into submission'; however, high-dose
chemotherapy may be very useful for the treatment of moderately resistant populations that are at a low tumour burden level.

A further corollary with respect to the log kill law is that drug resistance modulation may be disproportionately effective when combined
with high-dose chemotherapy. That is, modest changes in the value of β,
which would translate into only minor benefits when utilized with stan-
dard-dose chemotherapy, may generate substantial therapeutic effects
when employed with dose escalation. This is somewhat contrary to the
general impression that drug-resistance modulation techniques will
remove the necessity for high-dose treatments. Since drug-resistance
modulation is unlikely to restore complete drug sensitivity (or induced
hypersensitivity) then enhancement of high-dose effects may be a more
realistic objective.

7.5   Incompatibilities between the behaviour of clinical cancer and the random mutation model

There is certainly divided opinion as to how accurate the random mutation theory, which we have been emphasizing, is as a model for clinical
drug resistance. As discussed in a recent review (O'Brien and Cordon-
Cardo, 1991), there are at least two clinical phenomena that at first
examination do not appear to be easily reconciled with a basic 'mutation
to resistance' explanation for drug resistance. The first point that has
been made relates to the innate or constitutive patterns of drug sensitivity and resistance that are seen in various normal tissues. The most
sensitive tissue to most types of chemotherapy is clearly the normal
haematopoietic system. Next would appear to be the rapidly turning
over cells of the aerodigestive tract, with the upper gastrointestinal
tract (oral cavity, pharynx) being rather more sensitive to chemotherapy

effect than the colon. Other tissues that are characterized by regular cell turnover (skin, liver, pulmonary alveolar cells and renal tubular cells) tend to be sensitive to a few types of chemotherapeutic agent, but they are much less likely to constitute the dose-limiting tissue with most standard dose chemotherapy protocols.

Certain chemotherapeutic agents, such as doxorubicin, bleomycin and mitomycin C, produce organ-specific patterns of cumulative toxicity that appear to be only partly related to the capacity of these drugs to kill rapidly proliferating cells. Thus the nonproliferating muscle cells of the heart are subject to cumulative damage by agents such as doxorubicin; as a result, strict limits on the total dose of the drug have to be employed. This cardiac damage may manifest itself well before the problem of a tendency towards cumulative bone marrow damage begins to manifest itself.

Clearly, how a normal tissue responds to the toxic insult delivered by the various chemotherapeutic agents is partly a function of its cellular kinetic properties (its growth fraction, mean generation time, proportion of cells out of cycle, etc.) together with the constitutive expression of the various genes that are present in that particular tissue and the cell type. Cells of the gastrointestinal tract, the bone marrow and the lymphoid system seem to be particularly susceptible to apoptosis induction generated by genotoxic insult. Why this should be so is not entirely clear, although it is known that extensive apoptosis is a common physiological process in lymphoid tissue, presumably related to the elimination of cells that would cause immunological problems for the host. The haematopoietic cells share a common stem ancestor with lymphoid tissue and this may be one factor contributing to their relative propensity to undergo apoptosis under the influence of certain types of stress.

There does not appear to be a satisfactory understanding of the determinants of normal tissue response at this time. However, normal tissue resistance may not be directly relevant to the question of mutations to drug resistance in tumours. Whatever their initial relative sensitivity and resistance to anticancer agents, normal tissues do not tend to change this sensitivity despite repeated exposure to cytotoxic drugs. This issue was addressed in both Chapters 2 and 3, in which it was suggested that the normal cells appear to have little capacity to generate drug-resistant mutants, presumably because of their greater degree of fidelity of genetic replication.

The second phenomenon seemingly at variance with the random mutation model of drug resistance is sensitive relapse during clinical chemotherapy. What is meant by this term is the phenomenon that is seen with a few types of malignancy where, after a complete remission has been produced, the cancer recurs many months or even a few years later and still responds with almost the same degree of sensitivity as it displayed the first time (the operative word here is 'almost'). We observe this type of phenomenon usually in certain malignancies of lymphoid origin including Hodgkin's disease, so-called nodular lymphoma and, occasionally, in lymphoblastic leukaemia. In the case of Hodgkin's disease, the sensitive relapse is observed in approximately one half of patients whose cancer recurs more than a year following cessation of therapy. Those patients with recurrence in under a year have cancers that are nearly always quite resistant. The patients whose disease recurs at longer periods of time can, in 50% of instances, be put back into complete remission and, on occasion, be cured. The circumstance of repeated recurrence in what appears to be a predominantly drug-sensitive state is not uncommon with so-called nodular lymphoma, which is a less aggressive form of non-Hodgkin's lymphoma. One of the authors can recall from personal experience a patient who relapsed six times over a period of many years with disease that could still be put into remission with the same agents. Ultimately though, the patient developed complete refractoriness to therapy and this is generally what occurs with the other patients who display sensitive relapse.

It is important to remember that relapse in a drug-sensitive state is not the typical course that one sees with the vast majority of types of malignancy. Moreover, we are referring to the specific circumstance where a remission is induced by therapy and then treatment is discontinued. Disease that 'grows through' continuous treatment is, by definition, drug resistant.

Even though uncommon, the phenomenon of sensitive relapse is intriguing and does appear to be inconsistent with a simple model of selection for a drug-resistant population. The fact that a complete remission is initially produced with chemotherapy argues for an initial very high sensitive cell to resistant cell ratio. At this point, there are a number of scenarios that might occur. In the simplest case, we will have eliminated all of the drug-sensitive population and the drug-resistant clones will grow back, reconstitute the disease and be refractory to further treatment.

The second scenario would see an initial drug-sensitive population rather less sensitive than the average for the cohort of patients with this particular type of tumour but, nonetheless, sufficiently sensitive to allow a complete remission to be produced. In this case, however, there would still be a significant residual drug-sensitive population persisting after treatment is stopped. If the drug-sensitive cells have even a modest growth advantage in terms of shorter generation time or slightly higher probabilities of self-renewal, they will outgrow the resistant cells and regenerate a tumour that will still have a high sensitive-to-resistant cell ratio. After a further one or two courses of therapy generating further remissions, the resistant cell population will now dominate the recurrent disease so that further responses will not be seen.

The third possibility has to do with the production of so-called unstable resistance. This was mentioned briefly in Chapter 1 and again in Chapter 4, where we indicated that in most circumstances the effect of any sensitivity reversion rate can be ignored. However, this may well not be true for all situations. Some lines of tumour cells have the capacity, *in vitro* at least, to give rise at a low frequency to mutant cells that, in the absence of continuous selection, will rapidly revert to a drug-sensitive state.

The explanation of the molecular processes involved in this high reversion phenomenon is uncertain, but it has been suggested that it may be associated with drug-resistant states characterized by amplified gene segments present in extrachromosomal fragments. These fragments tend to segregate unequally at mitosis and may also become nonfunctional by other means. If the cells containing these chromosomal fragments are also characterized by slower growth rates than the sensitive cells (or other types of resistant cell) then they may paradoxically constitute a barrier to cure but at the same time not be sufficiently stable to grow out as a totally resistant population.

Indirect evidence suggesting that some type of unstable mutation may be playing a role in some of these sensitive relapse cases is illustrated by the unusual properties of the group of well-differentiated nodular lymphomas. These neoplasms tend to be very sensitive to chemotherapy, with nearly 100% complete remission rates being possible with multi-agent therapy. However, the tumour appears to be resistant to cure no matter how aggressively the chemotherapy is applied. Although some improvements in median survival have been noted with combination chemotherapy, long-term indefinite survivors are extremely rare and have probably not been significantly improved since the days of single agent treatment. These patients are also difficult to treat even using very high-dose chemotherapy and bone marrow transplantation.

One hypothetical model for this neoplasm would be that multidrug-resistant mutations are common in this tumour but tend to be unstable, at least in the earlier phases of the disease. Eventually a stable and highly resistant clone emerges, causing treatment failure.

There may be other explanations for the behaviour of these tumours but, at the present state of our knowledge, it would seem that mutations to resistance of an unstable nature provide one possibility. This would also suggest that the appropriate treatment strategy for these tumours would be either very-high-dose chemotherapy with marrow support or more intensive therapy with additional agents that do not share drug resistance pathways with the standard agents currently used. The availability in recent years of a number of new antilymphoma compounds that potentially are not cross-resistant with many of our standard agents should make it possible to test whether combinations of the appropriate number and type of drugs will finally be able to produce cures in these perplexing tumours.

7.6 Summary and conclusions

The issues raised in this chapter relate to whether the theoretical analysis of the process of drug-resistance evolution through mutations leads to any useful insights into clinical chemotherapy effects and if this, in turn, lends to new treatment strategies. Obviously the behaviour of malignancies is extremely complex and it is very unlikely that any relatively simple model will be able to explain every aspect of this behaviour. Nonetheless, the authors feel that there are a number of aspects of the response of clinical cancers to drugs that are consistent with the random mutation model of drug resistance and, indeed, are not easily explained by any other single set of assumptions.

Of these inferences, two in particular seem to emerge as being very generalizible. The first of these is the relationship between tumour burden (or age) and curability, and the second is the greatly increased potential for cure that is seen with multiagent therapy. It is true, as has been discussed earlier, that a model based on induced specific mutations would lead to some of the same conclusions. However, such a model would not distinguish between tumours of differing ages but of same size. Nor would an induction model provide any compelling rationale for molecular characterization of a tumour prior to commencement of therapy. If, for example, P-gp-negative B-cell lymphomas are 100% curable then there is no need to utilize an additional agent to modulate P-gp action. However, if it is known in advance that the tumour is P-gp positive then this will indicate a different strategy. It seems highly likely that as more is learned about the status of a tumour with respect to a whole range of drug resistance markers (e.g. MRP, p53, mutual *bcl-2* overexpression, etc.) this information will be utilized to construct more effective protocols. This is self-evident but it should be re-emphasized that a naive induction or kinetic model would provide no inherent rationale for measuring these particular parameters *prior* to treatment.

With respect to optimal sequencing of drugs it is conceded that the practical problems of utilizing true non-cross-resistant equivalent combinations may make this approach of very limited utility. Day's worst drug rule (1986) (see Chapter 6) would probably be easier to implement and evaluate but this would require a general willingness to undertake the appropriate clinical trials.

The approach of using very-high-dose chemotherapy with appropriate specialized support techniques (haemopoietic stem cell replacement etc.) can be justified by a variety of assumptions. However, the log kill law and the presumption of a spectrum of degrees of resistance in the target population do provide a sound theoretical basis for this practice.

As new classes of drug are developed that are designed to modulate oncogene and anti-oncogene effects, it is likely that new forms of scheduling and sequencing of drugs will be required. However, it is difficult not to believe that these new-generation compounds will, like current therapies, also be most effective against small tumour burdens.

References

Coldman, A.J., Coppin, C.M.L. and Goldie, J.H. (1988). Models for dose intensity. *Math. Biosci.*, 92: 97–113.

Coppin, C. (1987). The description of chemotherapy delivery: options and pitfalls. *Sem. Oncol.*, 14: 34–42.

Day, R.S. (1986). Treatment sequencing, asymmetry and uncertainty: new strategies for combining cancer treatments. *Cancer Res.*, 46: 3876–3885.

DeVita, V.T., Hubbard, S.M. and Longo, D.L. (1987). The chemotherapy of lymphomas: looking back and moving forward. *Cancer Res.*, 47: 5810–5824.

Fukuoka, M., Furuse, K., Sajo, N. *et al.* (1991). A randomised trial of cyclophosphamide, doxorubicin and vincristine versus cisplatin and etoposide versus alternatives of these regimens in small cell lung cancer. *J. Nat. Cancer Inst.*, 83: 855–861.

Hryniuk, W.M. and Bush, H. (1984). The importance of dose intensity of metastatic breast cancer. *J. Clin. Oncol.*, 2: 1281–1288.

Levin, L. and Hryniuk, W. (1987). The applications of dose intensity to problems in chemotherapy of ovarian carcinoma. *J. Clin. Oncol.*, 5: 756–767.

O'Brien, J.P. and Cordon-Cardo, C. (1991). On the origins of clinical drug resistance. *Sem. Cancer Biol.*, 2: 227–233.

Skipper, H. (1990). Dose intensity versus total dose of chemotherapy. An experimental basis. In *Important Advances in Oncology 1990*, ed. V.T. DeVita, S. Hellman and S.A. Rosenberg, pp. 43–64. Lippincott, Philadelphia.

Tannock, I.F., Boyd, N.F., Deboca, G. *et al.* (1988). A randomised trial of two dose levels of cyclophosphamide, methotrexate and fluorouracil chemotherapy for patients with metastatic breast cancer. *J. Clin. Oncol.*, 6: 1377–1387.

Further reading

DeVita, V.T. Jr (1993). Principles of chemotherapy in cancer. In *Principles and Practice of Oncology*, ed. R. Baserga, V.T. DeVita, S.A. Hellman and S.A. Rosenberg, pp. 276–292. Lippincott, Philadelphia, PA.

Fisher, R.J., Gaynor, E.R., Dahlberg, S. *et al.* (1993). Comparison of a standard regimen (CHOP) with three intensive chemotherapy regimens for advanced non-Hodgkin's lymphoma. *N. Eng. J. Med.*, 328: 1002–1006.

Gascoyne, R., Hoskins, P., Connors, J. *et al.* (1994a). A study of clinical and pathological variables affecting disease specific survival (DSS) of patients with diffuse large cell lymphoma treated with MACOP-B or VACOP-B. Uni-variate and multi-variate analysis. *Proc ASCO*, p. 1266.

Gascoyne, R., Tolcher, A., Coupland, R. *et al.* (1994b). The prognostic significance of immunophenotype in diffuse large cell lymphomas. *Modern Pathol.*, 7: A629.

Goldie, J.H. and Coldman, A.J. (1985). A model for tumour response to chemotherapy: an integration of the stem cell and random mutation hypothesis. *Cancer Invest.*, 3: 553–564.

Goldie, J.H. and Coldman, A.J. (1994). Arguments supporting the concept of non-cross resistant combinations of chemotherapy. *Cancer Invest.*, 12: 324–328.

Mead, C.M. and the International Germ Cell Cancer Collaborative Group (1995). *International Consensus Prognostic Classification for Metastatic Germ Cell Tumours Treated with Platinum Based Chemotherapy: A Final Report.* Proc. Asco IGCCCG.

Perry, M.C. (ed.) (1992). *The Chemotherapy Source Book.* Williams & Wilkins. Baltimore, MD.

van der Burg, M.E.L. *et al.* (1993). The effect of debulking surgery after induction chemotherapy on the prognosis of advanced epithelial cancer. *N. Eng. J. Med.,* 332: 629–634.

8

Directed versus random mutation and the problem of intrinsic resistance

8.1 Introduction

Much of this book has supported the notion that cancer cells resistant to anti-cancer drugs arise via random undirected mechanisms. The basis of this conclusion is not an exhaustive study of *in vivo* and *in vitro* tumour systems treated with all available drugs but a matter of generalization from a large body of evidence including the results of experiments of the fluctuation test type. As our review in Chapter 4 showed, a positive result in a fluctuation test implies that there exists a source of variation that cannot be attributed to the sampling variation expected under the directed mutation model. In terms of two possible processes that may result in resistance, directed mutation and random mutation, the fluctuation test can point to the existence of random mutation but not to the absence of directed mutation. Furthermore, since the essence of the fluctuation test is quantitative rather than qualitative, results from such experiments apply to the most common mechanism for the development of resistance under the experimental conditions. It is well known in cancer that many distinct genetic alterations can lead to resistance; as a result, the fluctuation test will provide information about the one that occurs most frequently (unless two or more mechanisms give rise to resistant cells with a similar frequency, in which case results will relate to the combination of these mechanisms).

8.2 The question of possible directed mutation in *E. coli*

Many investigators have considered the origin of resistant subtypes in different systems. In a paper in *Nature*, Cairns, Overbaugh and Miller (1988) discuss evidence for the existence of directed mutations in the

E. coli system. They present three lines of evidence that directed mutation exists: (a) several elements of a pathway for the influence of the
external environment on the incorporation of information into the DNA
are known to exist; (b) specific experiments show evidence, for some
systems, of the influence of the external environment upon the acquisition of altered phenotype; and (c) analysis of the frequency distributions
of the numbers of resistant cells displays variations from what would be
expected under the random mutation model. The experiments cited by
Cairns relate to lactose utilization by *E. coli* and are perhaps not directly
relevant to human cancer; however, the observation that directed mutations exist in one system raises the possibility that they exist in others.
Some of the techniques used by Cairns are of interest, in particular the
utilization of the frequency distribution of resistant cells, and potentially
provide methodologies that can be directly utilized in the analysis of
cancer data.

As discussed in Chapter 4, the distribution of the number of resistant
cells differs for the two hypotheses: directed mutation and random
mutation. The distribution is Poisson (at the time of exposure) for the
directed mutation model while the random time of creation of the progenitor resistant cells under the random mutation model lead to a different distribution (a *branching process* distribution). The nature of the
random mutation model is such that occasional 'jackpots' (large numbers which greatly exceed the average) of resistant cells are more likely
than under the directed mutation model. Indeed it is this phenomenon
that contributes to the larger variance between replicates in the random
mutation process than in the directed mutation process. Under the random mutation model, jackpots arise when a chance early transformation
to resistance produces large numbers of progeny by the time of exposure to the drug (Example 8.1 below). For a given average number of
resistant cells at the time of exposure to the drug, the random mutation
model predicts a much higher probability of substantially more than
average numbers of resistant cells in a single experiment than does
the directed mutation model. Using simple reasoning, it is possible to
derive formulae for the number of 'jackpots' under each model and we
will now show how this can be done.

For the directed mutation model, the number of resistant types, $R(N)$,
has a Poisson distribution so that the probability of obtaining r resistant
cells, $P\{R(N) = r\}$, when μ is the average number is given by (Equation
2.5), i.e.

$$P\{R(N) = r\} = \frac{[\mu]^r e^{-\mu}}{r!}. \tag{8.1}$$

(This formula holds for jackpots and nonjackpots alike.) The average number of induced resistant cells, μ is equal to ρN, where ρ is the directed mutation rate per unit cell (see Section 4.4) and N is the number of cells at drug exposure. In order to compare with an equivalent formula for the random mutation model, it is convenient to calculate the probability of a jackpot of at least r cells, i.e. $P\{R(N) \geq r\}$. A formula for this quantity may be obtained from Equation 8.1 by summing over all the possible states where there are r or more resistant cells. Numerically this is most simply done by summing all the probabilities of states with less than r resistant cells and subtracting this from unity, i.e.

$$P\{r(N) \geq r\} \geq 1 - \sum_{k=0}^{r-1} P\{R(N) = r\} = 1 - \sum_{k=0}^{r-1} \frac{\mu^k e^{-\mu}}{k!}. \tag{8.2}$$

A precise formula for the number of jackpots under the random mutation model is not easily obtained but an approximation can be obtained by observing that a jackpot is more likely to arise from a single early transition to resistance than by multiple, later transitions to resistance. This deduction is intuitively obvious to many writers and is frequently presented without further explanation; however, the authors do not find it that apparent and we will present an example which illustrates its justification.

Example 8.1

Consider a hypothetical tumour consisting of N' sensitive cells, which then undergoes five successive doublings (to $2N'$, $4N'$, $8N'$, $16N'$, $32N'$). Assume that the mean number of transitions is 0.0125 on the first doubling (i.e. $\alpha D' = 0.0125$) so that there are 0.025, 0.05, 0.1 and 0.2 transitions expected on each subsequent doubling. Now the expected number of resistant cells at the end from these transitions is given by the sum over the doublings of the expected number of transitions multiplied by their expected growth. For the first doubling this product is 0.2, being the expected number of transitions (0.0125) multiplied by the expected growth over the next four doublings ($\times 16$). Table 8.1 gives the calculations for subsequent doublings.

Table 8.1. *Numbers of transitions required and their probability to form a jackpot*

Tumour growth	No. cell divisions (D)	Mean No. transitions (αD)	Average No. resistant cells present at end arising from transitions	No. transitions required for jackpot (E) ($= 16 \times$ excess)	Normalized variate[a]	Probability of No. transitions E or greater
$N' \to 2N'$	N'	0.0125	0.2	1	8.8	1.2×10^{-2}
$2N' \to 4N'$	$2N'$	0.025	0.2	2	12.5	3.1×10^{-4}
$4N' \to 8N'$	$4N'$	0.05	0.2	4	17.7	2.4×10^{-7}
$8N' \to 16N'$	$8N'$	0.1	0.2	8	25.0	1.7×10^{-13}
$16N' \to 32N'$	$16N'$	0.2	0.2	16	35.3	3.1×10^{-25}
Overall: $N' \to 32N'$	$31N'$	0.3875	1.0	N/A	N/A	N/A

N/A, not applicable.
[a] $(E - \mu)/\sigma$ where $\mu = \alpha D$.

We see the expected pattern in that each doubling contributes the same expected number of resistant cells to the final total (i.e. 0.2). Overall we have that there are an expected 1.0 resistant cells present at the end of the experiment.

We will declare a jackpot when we observe many more resistant cells than the 1.0 expected. Let us define a jackpot in such an experiment to be an observation of 16 or more resistant cells. How can such jackpots arise? Qualitatively we might say that they can arise in the following ways:

- by an excess of transitions to resistance early in the experiment
- by an excess of transitions to resistance late in the experiment
- by some combination of early and late transitions.

The fifth column in Table 8.1 gives the number of transitions in each tumour doubling that would be sufficient, on their own, to produce a jackpot. Although the required number of transitions to produce a jackpot doubles with each tumour doubling so does the average number of transitions (column 3 in Table 8.1); as a result the ratio of these is constant. It is not immediately obvious whether excess early transitions are more likely to produce a jackpot than a corresponding number late in the growth of the tumour. In order to see whether excess early transitions are more likely than late transitions to yield jackpots we need to consider not just the mean but also the standard deviation of the number of transitions at each doubling. The standard deviation measures the variability about the mean so that the probability of obtaining a result, E, is dependent upon its distance from the mean, μ, measured in units of the standard deviation, σ, i.e.

$$\left| \frac{E - \mu}{\sigma} \right|.$$

The smaller this quantity the 'more likely' such a result, and conversely. The distribution of the number of transitions is Poisson so that $\sigma = \sqrt{\mu}$. In statistics $(E - \mu)/\sigma$ is frequently referred to as a *normalized variate*, since it has mean 0 and variance 1. The normalized values for the various extreme results at each doubling is given in column 6 of Table 8.1. As can be seen, this value increases as the tumour grows, indicating that jackpots are more likely to arise from a few early transitions. The final column of Table 8.1 shows the actual probability that a jackpot would arise from an excess of transitions at each doubling. This probability is only appreciable for the first doubling so that most jackpots will result from a single early transition.

We now return to the problem of finding an approximate formula for the probability of a jackpot under the random mutation model. The total number of resistant cells constituting a jackpot will consist of two broad lineages: those deriving from the first transition and those deriving from subsequent transformations. If we ignore those subsequently transformed (and their progeny) and consider the jackpot to consist solely of the ones resulting from the first transformation then we may infer the time at which the original clone came into existence as follows.

Let the (random) number of resistant cells be denoted by $R(N)$ when the tumour is of size N. Consider the case of a jackpot of $R(N) = r$ cells, which, we hypothesize, develops from a single early transition. If resistant and nonresistant cells grow at the same rate, then each cell present (both resistant and sensitive) at the time of the first transition must grow to form r progeny when the total tumour size is N (because the resistant cells do). Therefore, when the originating cell of the 'jackpot' transformed there were $N \div r$ cells in the total tumour. The probability that there is a jackpot of r resistant cells (among the total N cells) is equal to the probability that a single cell was transformed when the tumour was of size N/r. Here we must be a little careful since the likelihood that there will be a transformation at exactly that point is very small in a real tumour, which is continuously growing. However, if there is a transformation to resistance before this point (when the tumour is of size N/r) then there will be at least r resistant cells present at size N. This can be summarized in symbols by

$$P\{R(N) \geq r\} \geq$$
$$P\{\text{a first transformation occurs before tumour is of size } N/r\}. \quad (8.3)$$

The probability that there is a jackpot of r or more resistant cells is greater than or equal to the probability that a first transition to resistance occurs before the tumour is of size N/r.

The probability that a first transition occurs prior to N/r is equal to one minus the probability that no transition occurs prior to tumour size N/r. The distribution of the number of transitions occurring during the growth of a tumour from a single cell to N/r is Poisson with parameter $\mu = \alpha(N/r - 1)$. The required probability of no transitions is obtained from Equation 8.1 by substituting 0 for the value of r in this equation. This yields

$$P\{\text{no transformation occurs prior to } N/r\} = e^{-\alpha(N/r-1)}. \qquad (8.4)$$

From Equations 8.3 and 8.4 we obtain

$$P\{R(N) \geq r\} \geq 1 - e^{\alpha(N/r-1)}. \qquad (8.5)$$

If we now compare this to the earlier formula for the directed mutation model we are able to write this formula in terms of the average number of resistant cells μ (Equation 8.2). This was convenient since μ is observed whereas ρ must be inferred. It would be nice to use μ since it is observed in an experiment no matter which of the two models is operative. Now, as discussed in Chapter 5 under the random mutation model, the mean number of resistant cells is given by $\mu = \alpha N \ln(N)$ (Equation 5.18, p. 131). (In their development Cairns $et\ al.$ assumed $m = \alpha'N$, so that their formula for $P\{R(t) = r\}$ under the random mutation model does not include the $\ln(N)$ term.) Note the $\ln(N)$ term is different from the directed mutation model so that we have

$$\alpha = \frac{\mu}{N \ln(N)},$$

and we can replace α in Equation 8.5 by $\mu[N \ln(N)]$ to give

$$P\{R(t) \geq r\} \geq 1 - \exp\left(-\frac{\mu}{N \ln N}[N/r - 1]\right). \qquad (8.6)$$

In words, Equation 8.6 indicates that the probability of there being at least r resistant cells under the random mutation model exceeds the given formula.

Figure 8.1 gives some plotted values of the jackpot probabilities under the two models: Equation 8.5 for the random mutation model and Equation 8.6 for the directed mutation model. It can be seen that as the jackpot size increases the probability under the directed mutation model rapidly decreases whereas this decline is more gentle for the random mutation model, re-enforcing the point that jackpots are more likely under this scenario.

Cairns $et\ al.$ (1988) examined observed jackpot yields of $E.\ coli$ in lactose-containing environments and showed that they displayed functional forms which appeared midway between those predicted by the

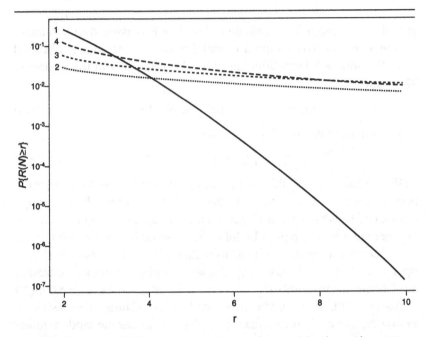

Fig. 8.1. Plots of $P\{R(N) \geq r\}$ versus r for the two models: directed mutation (Equation 8.2) and random mutation (Equations 8.6 and 8.7) for the case where a single resistant cell is expected, $\mu = 1$. For the directed mutation model (solid line 1), the probability of jackpots falls rapidly with increasing jackpot size. For the random model, the probability of a jackpot declines slowly with increasing size of jackpot. The shape of the relationship is not greatly affected by the resistant cell growth rate so that the shape is similar for equal growth rates (line 2), when the growth rate of resistant cells is slightly less (line 3: $\lambda_R/\lambda_S = 0.9$) and whehn substantially less (line 4: $\lambda_R/\lambda_S = 0.6$). As the relative growth rate of the resistant cells declines further, the formula (Equation 8.7) becomes less accurate, so that its shape for $\lambda_R/\lambda_S < 0.5$ is not obtainable from this equation. However we know that as the growth rate vanishes it must equal that for the directed model.

random mutation and directed mutation models. They hypothesized that this may have arisen because random mutation and directed mutation mechanisms were both operative, giving a hybrid relationship. The effect of having both mechanisms present is to take a weighted sum of the curves (in Fig. 8.1) for the directed and random mutation processes with the appropriate parameter values ρ and α. The net effect is that most jackpots will derive from the random mutational process since it has a much greater probability of leading to a jackpot for values of ρ and α that are of the same magnitude.

However, it is also pertinent to ask whether there are other potential explanations of a distribution with a form midway between the form for the directed mutation model and the form for the random mutation model. In fact, there is one simple assumption we made in deriving the distribution of the number of jackpots under the random mutation model that if not true must give a form which is between the directed mutation and the random mutation forms. This assumption was that the resistant cells grow at the same rate as the drug-sensitive cells. If this assumption is not true then the distribution of jackpots under the random mutation model is altered, although unchanged under the directed mutation model.

A simple thought experiment will illustrate the dependence of jackpot probabilities upon growth rate. Consider a random mutation model in which the newly created resistant cells possess no capacity to divide. If each resistant cell, once created, persists to the conclusion of the experiment then the number of resistant cells at termination is equal to the number of cells that transform from sensitivity to resistance. The distribution of resistant cells at the conclusion of the experiment is equal to the distribution of total number of transformations from sensitivity to resistance prior to drug exposure. This distribution has a Poisson form where the mean number of transformations is given by αN. (This can be contrasted with the mean number of resistant cells when growth is the same as that of the drug-sensitive cells of $\mu = \alpha N \ln(N)$; this higher value reflects the effect of growth of transformed resistant cells.) When there is no resistant cell replication, the jackpot distribution will follow a Poisson distribution whereas when growth is the same as sensitive cells it will be of the form previously given. If resistant cells do grow at a rate that is less than that of sensitive cells then their resulting distribution will look more like a mix between a Poisson and random mutation distribution. A formula for probability of a jackpot of size r under the random mutation model in the case where sensitive and resistant cells grow at different rates can be developed using the same steps as were used to derive Equation 8.6. (Unfortunately the approximation used in deriving the formulae, that jackpots principally result from early transitions, becomes less accurate as the growth rate of the resistant cells slows.) Since no further insight is provided by the derivation of this formula we merely state it here:

$$P\{R(N) \geq r\} \geq 1 - \exp\left(-\frac{\mu(1 - \lambda_R/\lambda_S)}{[N - N^{\lambda_R/\lambda_S}]}\left[\frac{N}{r^{\lambda_S/\lambda_R}} - 1\right]\right) \qquad (8.7)$$

where λ_S and λ_R are the growth parameters of the sensitive and resistant cells, respectively. When the growth rates are equal, Equation 8.7 reduces to the formula in Equation 8.6. Previously we have indicated (see Example 8.1) that jackpots, when observed, are more likely to result from the effect of a single early transition. In this case the $\geq$ sign in Equation 8.6 can be replaced by $=$ since other sources of jackpot are negligible. As resistant cell growth slows, early transitions will contribute proportionately less to the total of resistant cells and early transitions are less likely to be the source of observed jackpots. In the mathematical limit where resistant cells do not grow at all, the distribution of resistant cells is equal to the distribution of transitions (which is Poisson). In cases of slow resistant cell growth ($\lambda_R < \lambda_S$) multiple late transitions are more likely to be a cause of a jackpot than single early transitions. In these circumstances the $\geq$ sign in Equation 8.7 is more like $>$ and the equation is not very helpful. Equation 8.7 is plotted in Fig. 8.1 for values of the ratio λ_R/λ_S for which it is likely to be accurate ($\lambda_R/\lambda_S > 0.5$). It can be seen that for the range of values of λ_R/λ_S between 1.0 and 0.5 there is not much difference in predicting probabilities of a jackpot. Nevertheless, we know that as the growth rate of the resistant cells slows in comparison with that of the sensitive cells the distribution of jackpots must approach that of a Poisson distribution.

The assertion of the existence of directed mutation has been challenged by others (Lenski and Mittler, 1993). They discuss alternative origins for excess numbers of appropriate E. coli when grown in a selecting environment and indicate how departures from various assumptions can result in findings seemingly at variance with a random mutation hypothesis. Much of their discussion is specific to experiments conducted in E. coli and will not be presented here, although it does serve to illustrate that detailed knowledge of the behaviour of cells in different milieu is necessary in order to draw conclusions about the mechanisms of resistance development.

Clearly whether adaptation can occur in a directed fashion is a fundamental question for biology, but what bearing does it have on cancer chemotherapy? Although each model postulates different underlying mechanisms, do they make distinct predictions for the effects of cancer chemotherapy? Many of the predicted relationships for each model are the same. An area where they differ is in the influence of the 'history' of the tumour on the observed distribution of resistant cells. Because resistant cells can arise at any point during the lifetime of the tumour, the growth history influences the final distribution of resistant cells for the random model. This would not happen under the directed mutation model unless events in the history affected the susceptibility of succeeding generations of cells to have resistance 'induced'. A further difference is that large numbers of resistant cells are more likely under the random mutation model (although still rare) than under the directed mutation model. The random mutation model predicts that completely resistant tumours will be more common than they would be for the directed mutation model (given identical overall average results).

8.3   Resistance associated with the three-dimensional configuration of experimental tumours

Teicher *et al.* (1990) and Kobayashi *et al.* (1993) have described experiments with mouse EMT-6 cells in which exposure to antineoplastic agents resulted in a measurable change in the three-dimensional structure of the tumour mass, which was associated with an alteration in sensitivity to cytotoxic drugs.

The EMT-6 cells can be grown as solid tumours either in the whole animal or in tissue culture. In the latter they form multicellular spheroids, aggregates of tumour cells numbering from a few thousand to many millions of cells that grow in a semisolid culture medium as nearly spherical discrete masses Studies on these spheroids indicate that, superficially at least, they resemble the structure of *in vivo* tumours, which also frequently grow as near spherical masses. The exterior shell of the spheroid is made up of rapidly dividing cells and on penetrating deeper into the spheroid the proportion of dividing cells diminishes; the central part of the larger spheroids is made up of necrotic cell debris.

When exposed to cytotoxic drug *in vitro*, the rapidly proliferating cells on the rim of the spheroid are killed off, exposing the deeper layer cells, which now begin to proliferate more quickly. Repeated exposure to sublethal concentrations of a variety of cytotoxic agents results in a distinct change in the physical shape of the cells constituting the spheroid. Whereas prior to chemotherapeutic exposure the cells in the spheroid tend to be relatively loosely aggregated, when the spheroids start to display resistance to cytotoxic agents they appear to be much more densely packed together and there is some evidence that there are now more actual cell-to-cell connections in these resistant tumour cells. If these resistant spheroids are then disaggregated into two-dimensional monolayers of cells and treated with cytotoxic agents, they display little or no drug resistance. In these experimental systems, therefore, there is no doubt that drug resistance is strongly associated with the three-dimensional configuration that the tumour cells display and that this resistance is lost when cells are dispersed and are no longer in close contact with each other.

There are a number of interesting questions that arise from these studies. The first is whether this is a laboratory artefact confined to a few atypical cell lines or whether this is a more general phenomenon.

The second question is whether this constitutes an 'induced' phenomenon or is it caused by random mutation of an unusual phenotype that is only able to express its resistance under certain conditions. In other words, the cell lines that show resistance in the spheroid form and sensitivity in a monolayer may be a genetic variant that has been selected for by the conditions of the experiment.

Part of the mechanism of resistance in this system appears to be the capacity of the resistant cells to produce intercellular bridges, which enable significant direct communication among the cells making up the spheroid. This could, in theory, allow the transmission of resistance-mediating elements from one cell to another. This still leaves open the question raised in the preceding paragraph, namely, is this property an epigenetic induced phenomenon or is it the expression of a complex phenotype that has arisen through spontaneous mutation?

8.4   Induction of drug-resistant gene expression by chemotherapeutic stress

Chaudhary and Roninson (1993), have described apparent directed mutation phenomena in a number of lines of human malignant cells exposed to a variety of cytotoxic agents. In these experiments, different human cell lines were exposed *in vitro* to cytotoxic concentrations of drugs such as ara-C and hydroxyurea. In a number of the lines tested (but not all) a proportion of the cells in the treated population showed increased expression of *mdr-1*, as demonstrated by increased messenger RNA for P-gp and for increased P-gp expression in the cell itself. This occurred in approximately 5% of the treated cells and was manifested only after the individual cells began to show gross morphological evidence of cytotoxic damage.

What was of unusual interest in these experiments was that the increased expression of *mdr-1* persisted for a sustained period of time after withdrawal of the cytotoxic agent. In other words, the increased P-gp persisted through several rounds of cell division and appeared to represent the directed mutation of a heritable property in the malignant cells. This was not a specific directed mutation of resistance mechanisms related to the toxic drug itself but appeared to be more consistent with a general response phenomenon by the cells to an environmental stress. This would be easily understood if this was an upregulated response confined to the cells that had been directly exposed to the cytotoxic agent. However, the apparent persistence of the phenomenon after drug withdrawal and after cell division indicates that in some cells the stress 'imprinted' itself and persisted for an extended period of time. As the authors pointed out, this is does not necessarily imply a change in expression at the level of the gene but could represent some type of persisting change in the processing of the messenger RNA resulting in an extended half life and greater amounts of P-gp being synthesized.

Clearly this provocative result needs to be explored further, including the performance of experiments that would rigorously exclude random mutation processes which might underlie it. For instance, the authors did report that a very small proportion of the untreated cells appeared to overexpress *mdr-1* constitutively and one would need to exclude experimental conditions that could result in an enrichment of this basal population to form the progenitors of the cells that were observed after drug withdrawal. In this context both ara-C and hydroxyurea interfere directly with DNA synthesis and could function as mutagenic agents. Such effects could make it difficult, even within the context of a fluctuation test, to distinguish readily between induced and spontaneous events.

8.5 Drug resistance resulting from epigenetic phenomena

It has been suggested (see review by Nyce, 1997) that instances of acquired drug resistance may be associated with toxic stress-induced methylation or demethylation of a variety of genes that can mediate drug resistance. Methylation of genes is a crucially important process that regulates the selective expression or silencing of gene function. It is a key component of embryonic development (and cellular differentiation generally) where genes are switched on or off in a complex and specific order.

Alterations in gene methylation can be observed in cells that survive cytotoxic drug exposure, suggesting a mechanism for rapidly inducing phenotypic changes in cells. Nyce postulates an epigenetically unstable state in which nonlethally damaged cells respond by randomly methylating (or demethylating) regions of their genome. As these epigenetic changes may persist for at least five rounds of cell division, altered (and presumably drug-resistant) cells will be observed on tumour regrowth.

There are some problems with this hypothesis (at least in its current state of development), but clearly further investigation needs to be done to clarify the role that methylation plays in acquired drug resistance.

If the methylation process is truly random then it is difficult to see why the cells produced are necessarily more drug resistant than their ancestors. Resistance-mediating genes may be just as likely to be suppressed as activated by a random methylation process. This would be true for sensitivity-mediating genes as well. For that matter, oncogenes that are critically required for maintenance of the malignant phenotype might be silenced, resulting in spontaneous apoptosis or reversion to a more normal phenotype.

If only changes in one direction (more resistance) are produced then the theory starts to resemble directed mutation. It should be recalled that a single exposure to a cytotoxic drug acting in a directed fashion would not necessarily be selective, as no preadaptation is assumed.

Likewise, the mechanism of epigenetic instability in cancer needs to be explained as well as why drug resistance through methylation–demethylation apparently does not occur in normal cells, where we might simplistically assume that it would be highly probable. That is, such a fine-tuned adaptation technique would appear to have great survival advantage.

The whole question of the role of epigenetic processes such as methylation needs further study. Random gene changes induced by this method would behave like directed mutations in experiments of the fluctuation test type; that is, unless one postulated that there was a pre-existing genetic disposition for certain DNA sites to become methylated during times of cytotoxic drug exposure. That would in a sense, however, reduce the argument to a variation of genetic preadaptation.

8.6   The development of high levels of resistance

It is a common, but not universal, observation that resistant cells may divide at the same or slightly lower rates than their parental lines in a 'normal' environment. Such a phenomenon is understandable from an evolutionary perspective since this is precisely how the parental line achieved dominance. Parental lines also have to be resistant to toxins commonly found in their normal environment; however we (in our discussion on resistance) are concerned with the spontaneous introduction of uncommon toxins in order to achieve a therapeutic result. Tumours, and in particular spontaneous human tumours, have generally not gone through such a selection mechanism and so the cells which make up these tumours have not been selected for their fitness. It is, therefore, not impossible to conceive that nonlethal mutations occurring in these cells have a greater *de novo* likelihood to provide competitive advantage than would be the case in more established systems. For example, gene amplification can provide resistance by offering an expanded target for any drugs attempting to block protein synthesis. In the nonselective medium it provides a potential for enhanced protein synthesis and possible growth advantage. Observations from repeatedly passaged tumour cell lines will not provide definitive information on the growth rates of resistant variants in spontaneous tumours since the repeat passaging of such lines will tend to select for fast-growing parent populations. Indeed several experimental systems are extremely resistant to some forms of chemotherapy, implying that some resistant cells can grow faster than sensitive variants. We will explore here what the effect of modest growth advantages to resistant cells can be on the development of resistance in the random mutation model.

We may use the approach presented in Section 6.2 to develop equations that give the mean number of resistant cells as a function of the overall tumour size. However, because we are now assuming that sensitive and resistant cells grow at different rates, it is necessary to have different growth parameters for each compartment. For simplicity, we will only consider the case where cells grow exponentially. Assuming that sensitive and resistant cells divide at rates b_S and b_R and spontaneously die at rates d_S and d_R then the net growth rate of each compartment is given by $\lambda_S = (b_S - d_S)$ and $\lambda_R = (b_R - d_R)$, respectively. New transitions from sensitivity to resistance will occur at rates αb_S per cell as before (Equation 6.1). Assuming that the tumour starts from a single sensitive cell then the number of sensitive cells, $S(t)$, at time t is given by

$$S(t) = \exp\{(\lambda_S - \alpha b_S)t\}. \tag{8.8}$$

which is the same equation as before. We have used the more accurate formula $\lambda_S - \alpha b_S$ rather than λ_S (as suggested in the discussion following Equation 6.1) since we may consider situations where αb_S is not much smaller than λ_S. Substituting Equation 8.8 into Equation 6.1 and replacing the term $\lambda R(t)$ in this equation with $\lambda_R R(t)$ provides a new equation for $R(t)$. Solving this equation yields:

$$R(t) = \alpha b_S \exp\{\lambda_R t\} \frac{[1 - \exp\{(\lambda_S - \alpha b_S - \lambda_R)t\}]}{[\lambda_S - \alpha b_S - \lambda_R]}. \tag{8.9}$$

Because $R(t)$ has a somewhat more complex form than before, $N(t) = S(t) + R(t)$ is no longer a single exponential and it is not so easy to express the number of resistant cells as a function of the overall tumour size, i.e. $R(N)$. Therefore, it is necessary to make calculations at various values of t and then sum $S(t)$ and $R(t)$ to yield $N(t)$. In this way R may be calculated as a function of N. Some example calculations are presented in Table 8.2. In this case the parameters have been chosen so that the resistant cells grow 20% faster than the sensitive cells and the doubling time of the tumour is 20 times that of the interdivision times of the cells. There are two distinct ways in which stem cells may grow at different rates in the compartment model: the birth (division) rates may differ or the death (apoptosis) rates may differ (or some combination of the two). Measured division rates seem to show less variation than apoptosis rates so we have assumed that $b_S = b_R$ but d_S and d_R differ. The scale of measurement of t (i.e. hours, days, weeks, etc.) affects the absolute values of the birth and death parameters; their relative size (b/d) reflects the balance between division and apoptosis. For simplicity, it is assumed that t is measured on a scale in which $b_S = 1$. These assumptions resulted in the following parameter values: $b_S = b_R = 1.0$, $d_S = 0.95$ and $d_R = 0.94$. For this calculation $\alpha = 10^{-5}$. Examination of Table 8.2 shows that the effect of the modest increase in the growth rate of the resistant cells compared with the sensitive cells becomes quickly apparent so that at 10^6 cells 1 in 100 is resistant. By the time that there are 10^{10} cells 1 in 10 is resistant. The final column of the table provides the same proportion for a tumour in which there is no growth advantage and no loss. It can be seen that by the time a tumour reaches 10^{10} cells,

Table 8.2. *Expected number of resistant cells when the growth rate of resistant cells is 20% greater than that of the sensitive cells and for which* $\alpha = 10^{-5}$

Size of tumour	No. resistant cells	Proportion of cells resistant	Proportion when growth is same as sensitive cells
10^3	3	3×10^{-3}	6.9×10^{-5}
10^4	53	5.3×10^{-3}	9.2×10^{-5}
10^5	890	8.9×10^{-3}	1.2×10^{-4}
10^6	1.4×10^4	1.4×10^{-2}	1.4×10^{-4}
10^7	2.4×10^5	2.4×10^{-2}	1.6×10^{-4}
10^8	3.7×10^6	3.7×10^{-2}	1.8×10^{-4}
10^9	5.8×10^7	5.8×10^{-2}	2.1×10^{-4}
10^{10}	9.0×10^8	9.0×10^{-2}	2.3×10^{-4}

the effect of spontaneous cell death coupled with a modest growth advantage of the resistant cells can combine to provide an approximate 400-fold increase in the expected number of resistant cells.

The above phenomenon is also reflected in the probability of jackpot probabilities. One way to see this is to compare the sizes of jackpots with the same probability for the same value of α but different growth rates. This can be done using a variant of Equation 8.9 where we replace μ by its expected value given α and N.

8.7   Summary and conclusions

We have briefly reviewed some of the experimental data that might be interpreted as suggesting an induced or directed mutation process as being one mechanism of forming drug-resistant cells. Although the issue is clearly complex the authors feel that no compelling evidence has been presented to date that would suggest that spontaneous mutations are not the dominant process involved in generating drug-resistant phenotypes.

Demonstrations of specific resistant mutations could have enormous scientific and philosophical complications, well beyond that of the issue of cancer treatment. However, the neo-Darwinist view still appears to be the correct one. Although the transmission of cultural information from one human generation to the next appears to be directed, Nature seems to prefer the random transmission of information at the genetic level.

The discussion in Section 8.6 illustrates how the rather large increases in the proportions of resistant cells can be achieved by modest alterations in parameter values for the growth of resistant cells and a general process of cell birth and nonselective cell loss. Extremely high proportions of resistant cells can be generated (~1 in 10) in tumours of clinical dimensions by having resistant cells grow somewhat faster (20%) in a tumour experiencing cell loss in the ranges that seem consistent with observation. Such an expansion of resistance is provided by the magnifying lens of growth after transition and would not occur in a directed model.

References

Cairns, J. Overbaugh, J. and Miller, S. (1988). The origin of mutants. *Nature*, 335: 142–145.

Chaudhary, P.M. and Roninson, I.B. (1993). Induction of multi-drug resistance in human cells by transient exposure to different chemotherapeutic agents. *J. Nat. Cancer Inst.*, 85: 632–639.

Kobayashi, H., Man, S., Graham, C.H. *et al.* (1993). Acquired multi-cellular mediated resistance to alkylating agents in cancer. *Proc. Natl. Acad. Sci. USA: Cell Biol.*, 90: 3294–3298.

Lenski, R.E. and Mittler, J.E. (1993). The directed mutation controversy and reo-Darwinism. *Science*, 259: 188–194.

Nyce, J.W. (1997). Drug induced DNA hypermethylation: a potential mediator of acquired drug resistance during cancer chemotherapy. *Mutat. Res.*, 386: 1531–1561.

Teicher, B.A., Herman, T.S., Holden, S.A. *et al.* (1990). Tumour resistance to alkylating agents conferred by mechanisms operative only *in vitro*. *Science*, 247: 1457–1461.

Further reading

Bennet, D.C. (1985). *Darwin's Dangerous Idea*. Simon & Schuster, New York. A thoughtful popular account of the nature of Darwinian evolution.

Chen, G., Jaffrezou, J.P., Fleming, W.H. *et al.* (1994). Prevalence of multi-drug resistance related to activation of the *mdr-1* gene in tumour sarcoma mutants derived by single step doxorubicin selection. *Cancer Res.*, 54: 4980–4987.

Goldie, J.H. and Coldman, A.J. (1983). Quantitative model for multiple levels of drug resistance in clinical tumours. *Cancer Treat. Rep.*, 67: 923–931.

Hoffman, R.M. (1994). The three dimensional question – can clinically relevant tumour drug resistance be measured *in vitro? Cancer Metastasis Rev.*, 13: 160–173.

Jaffrezou, J.P., Chen, G., Duran, G.E. *et al.* (1994). Mutation rates and mechanisms of resistance to etoposide determined from fluctuation analysis. *J. Nat. Cancer Inst.*, 86: 1152–1158.

9

Some final thoughts on the problem of drug resistance

9.1 Introduction

Analysis of the process of drug resistance indicates that it appears to be only too easy for malignancies to generate many varieties of drug-resistance mechanisms. Once a tumour has reached a certain critical size a combination of large numbers of candidate cells together with genetic instability will ensure that the collective molecular heterogeneity of the neoplasm will be immense. In retrospect, the surprising thing is not that cancers are difficult to treat with drugs but that some are highly sensitive to drug therapy and indeed are potentially curable. Although the addition of new cytotoxic agents provides a reasonably steady incremental improvement in cancer therapy outcome, these increments are small and are for the most part confined to the classes of tumour that are known already to be drug responsive. Malignancies such as pancreatic carcinoma, renal cell cancer, melanoma and non-small cell lung cancer are only minimally responsive to cytotoxic agents and it seems unlikely that random drug searches will yield single agents that are going to be much more effective than the drugs we currently possess. A major problem with these types of cancer seems to be the large number of different multidrug resistant mechanisms that they express. Modulation of one or two of these mechanisms is unlikely to be sufficient to render the advanced forms of the tumour curable. The greater the number of discreet mechanisms that need to be disabled then, of course, the more logistically cumbersome the treatment protocol becomes. Moreover, resistance-modulating drugs will be subject to the same problems associated with tumour heterogeneity as are the standard cytotoxic agents: variant cells that express proteins which are less susceptible to modulation or have altered transport of the modulating drugs across cell membranes will be selected for by the treatment process.

238

The cellular and molecular heterogeneity displayed by malignant tumours would suggest that there will always be a risk that treatment failure will occur because of the presence of a malignant subclone that possesses properties which allow it to survive therapy. This risk can be reduced by applying treatment when the tumour is still early in its growth history and when the total number of cells to be eliminated is small. A critical additional factor will be the requirement to utilize therapeutic programmes that are directed against molecular abnormalities which are specific to the individual cancer that is being treated. This approach will require the full range of molecular probes that are currently being employed in research programmes being utilized for clinical diagnostic purposes.

Precise molecular diagnosis on its own will not yield superior treatment outcomes; it needs to be integrated with a drug development programme that concentrates on producing specific inhibitors or agonists for the disregulated gene products that are associated with the malignant state.

Up till now, the pattern seen in identifying new drugs for oncology has been for preclinical scientists to develop a novel cytotoxic compound and then for clinical investigators to search for a class of tumour that is sensitive to the new agent. This is an expensive, time-consuming process in which disappointing results far outnumber successes. The availability of ever more drugs and at least some moderately effective protocols makes progress more rather than less difficult. Ethical considerations operate to restrict new drug evaluations to patients with known drug-resistant disease, making it correspondingly harder to assess new approaches for previously untreated patients.

It seems to the authors that the sequence of 'find a drug, then look for a disease' will need to be reversed. A more rational strategy is surely to exploit our increasing ability to make precise molecular diagnoses and then to utilize drug combinations where the composition is dictated by the properties of the individual patient's malignancy itself. This will require examining the whole process whereby new treatments are assessed and then licensed. The present sytem is predicated largely on the assumption that single agents, 'magic bullets', will be found for whole classes of tumour. Our experience to-date with cytotoxic agents suggests that this is unlikely to be the case.

9.2   The role of oncogenes in mediating drug resistance

The realization (based on observations made in the period 1986–96) that a number of the genes which are directly involved with the production of the neoplastic state in the cell are at the same time significant mediators of anticancer drug resistance must rank as one of the most important discoveries in cancer biology in recent years. This fact, together with the known genetic instability of malignant cells, goes some distance towards explaining the virtual invariable association of malignancy with the capacity to develop drug resistance.

There are many types of genetic change that can mediate drug resistance and a number of these have been mentioned in this text. However, it appears that some of the most important ones may be the same mutations that lead to malignancy in the first place. Dysfunction of oncogenes or anti-oncogenes commonly appears to result in diminished sensitivity to standard cytotoxic drugs. However, it is not clear whether this is true for all of the family of cancer-inducing genes. Overexpression of the c-*myc* oncogene can on its own actually sensitize the tumour cell to apoptosis induction. Other examples no doubt exist, though the behaviour of most clinical cancers suggests that configurations of oncogenes and tumour suppressor genes which lead to drug hypersensitivity are uncommon.

One of the intriguing questions relating to drug resistance is the relative contribution made by the 'cancer-inducing genes' compared with that made by the large number of genes that affect individual drug action (the 'traditional' drug-resistance genes, as it were). Since the subset of drug-curable malignancies must also have cancer gene abnormalities, it is apparent that these need not be sufficient to produce high levels of drug resistance. Presumably the least favourable circumstances will be those in which there is both considerable oncogene dysregulation and many types of multidrug-resistant mutation. We can speculate that one reason why cancers arising in later life tend to be more drug-resistant than paediatric cancers may be related to the number of mutations that occur prior to the 'creation' of the malignant clone. The differences in elapsed time between the first cancer mutation and the final step providing clonal expansion would suggest that many more mutations are involved in the generation of cancer arising in the elderly. Undoubtedly other factors will also be contributory.

We have been emphasizing in this book how certain mathematical approaches can provide insights into the nature of the drug-resistance process. Fluctuation type tests for drug resistance are predicated on the assumption that the drug-resistant mutations arise after the malignant transformation has occurred. However, these fluctuations will not be apparent with respect to any drug-resistant mechanisms that are part of the transformation process itself. These mechanisms will be present in all (or nearly all) of the cells making up the malignant clone and hence will provide the 'background' level of resistance of the tumour upon which further drug-resistant mutations will arise. The mutations leading to the malignant state will, in effect, provide the true basal level of intrinsic resistance of the cancer, which will then be further modified by subsequent mutations.

The fact that cancer-inducing genes can in themselves lead to drug resistance would appear to make the job of the therapist even more difficult than it is. However, we might suggest that it is not unrealistic to expect that exploitation of this knowledge has great potential for significantly improving the results of systemic cancer therapy. In fact, we are tempted to say that if efficient abrogation of the function of the dysregulated cancer-inducing genes does not provide more effective therapy then it becomes very difficult to imagine what effective therapy *will* require.

The outline of what may comprise systemic cancer therapy at the turn of the century is beginning to take shape. It seems very likely that these treatment programs will consist of various modulators or inhibitors of dysregulated gene function combined with a variety of standard older cytotoxic agents. In addition, antihormones and antigrowth factor compounds of various types will almost certainly be utilized.

It remains, at present, only an optimistic hope that such specialized forms of combination chemotherapy will truly constitute an advance over existing approaches. There are, however, tantalizing hints from preliminary experimental studies that suggest that this may indeed be possible. This field will open up a whole new area of anticancer agent pharmacology and no doubt new principles of treatment optimization will need to be developed.

9.3   Cancer therapy in the 21st century

It seems more than likely that lessons that have been learned from cytotoxic agent treatment of cancer will still apply to more exotic and sophisticated therapies: small and/or early tumour burdens will be much more readily curable than will advanced disease and an initial unsuccessful strategy will make things significantly more difficult when a re-treatment manoeuvre is carried out.

There are a number of questions that will need to be addressed as we move into the next era of systemic therapy of cancer. To begin with, we will need to know which of the dysregulated genes in a particular tumour represent the most vulnerable therapeutic targets. Many cancers by the time they are clinically apparent appear to have several genetic lesions in their growth-signalling pathways, their cell cycle-promoting genes and in the genes that directly regulate apoptosis. Will there be any preferential group of genes that need to be targeted when developing therapy? Will it matter, for instance, if a particular mutation appears to be one that has evolved very early in the generation of the neoplastic clone (e.g. p53 mutation in Li–Fraumeni syndrome tumours) or is it genetic changes that have evolved later in the evolution of the fully malignant clone (e.g. telomerase activation) that will prove to be the sensitive 'choke points' for inhibiting tumour growth?

Will it be more effective to abrogate simultaneously more than one dysregulated gene function or will some complex sequencing of the deleted functions be more effective in terminating tumour growth? Will it be more effective to inhibit the function of two genes that are acting on similar pathways (e.g. *bcl-2* overexpression and mutatated *Rb* gene function) or will it prove more useful to block a growth signal transduction gene (mutated *ras*) together with inhibiting overexpression of *bcl-2*? Will particular treatment strategies be highly tumour specific or even individual patient specific?

Most of the studies reported to date have simply examined the consequences of inhibition of one oncogene in a tumour cell line together with some other type of therapeutic agent, e.g. corticosteroids or alkylating agents. It is of great interest to note that *in vitro*, and at least to some degree *in vivo* as well, inhibiting one of the important oncogenes in a tumour cell line may be sufficient on its own to cause reversion to a normal or at least nonmalignant phenotype and to increase cytotoxic drug sensitivity dramatically. We should, however, remember that we already have many effective forms of therapy for *in vitro* cell lines and for transplanted tumours. It may be overly optimistic to expect that an advanced clinical tumour can be effectively dealt with by a single gene function abrogation. This might be the case, but it seems more probable that multiple pathways will need to be inhibited to ensure eradication of a malignant clone. Determining these strategic approaches will be a challenging and fascinating area of cancer research.

If, as it seems likely, standard cytotoxic agents and radiation will be needed to enhance cell-killing effects, it will be important to determine if combinations of cytotoxic agents will be more effective than a single agent given at maximum tolerated dose. We would suspect that the combination will probably prove to be the more effective but the rules of the game may turn out to be different under circumstances where major channels leading to apoptosis are opened up and the goal becomes one of maximizing the log kill effect by dose escalation.

Will antisense nucleic acids prove to be the optimal agents for gene inhibition or will small-molecular-weight compounds (i.e. standard drugs) turn out to be the more useful if they can be made specific in their binding to the active sites of oncoproteins? On the one hand, antisense compounds have the advantage that they can be made to almost any desired degree of specificity. Moreover, a series of such compounds can be produced so that they will probably affect all of the common mutant forms of the messenger RNA that they are required to bind with. On the other hand, small-molecular-weight compounds have the advantage of ease of administration and the feasibility of being given in saturation doses. Whether they can be made specific enough to have appropriate therapeutic indices is an unanswered question at this time.

9.3   New forms of drug resistance

A final question that comes to mind returns to the central issue that we have been dealing with in this text. This is the enormous capacity of neoplastic cell populations to generate diverse forms, some of which will be expected to have an enhanced capacity for survival under various selecting environments.

We have seen how readily cancer cells evolve multiple pathways of resistance to standard cytotoxic agents with the result that it becomes impossible to cure most advanced tumours with any realistic number of cytotoxic drugs. When actual clinical tumours are being treated with compounds for deleting gene growth functions or suppressing anti-apoptosis gene effects, we will need to know whether the cell can evolve new and exotic growth pathways that will allow them to evade specific antigene therapy. To put the question in Darwinian terms, is

244 Drug resistance in cancer

there present within any advanced neoplastic cell population a very small number of tumour cells that by chance have become equipped with very unusual signal transduction and cell cycle control elements that will allow them to escape efficient shutting down of *bcl-2* production combined with massive drug-induced DNA damage?

We suspect that the answer to this last question will be both yes and no. Some malignancies that hitherto have proved very difficult to treat with conventional cytotoxic agents and radiation will probably prove vulnerable to more sophisticated forms of therapy. There will probably also be other types of malignancy that will show evidence of novel means for maintaining their growth advantage despite the loss of several critical functioning genetic components. The challenge then will be to identify what these more exotic and obscure pathways are and to begin to chart the strategies for dealing with them. In the meantime, though, the 'yardsticks'[†] will have been moved forward and we can with cautious optimism expect that both the number and the proportion of treatment-resistant neoplasms will have been substantially reduced.

[†] A North American football term that determines the minimum amount of ground that must be gained in the next series of plays. The object is to move the yardsticks ever closer to the opponents' goal line.

Index